FOOD VALUES
Calcium

FOOD VALUES

Calcium

Leah Wallach

PERENNIAL LIBRARY

Harper & Row, Publishers, New York
Cambridge, Philadelphia, San Francisco
London, Mexico City, São Paulo, Singapore, Sydney

FOOD VALUES: CALCIUM. Copyright © 1989 by Harper & Row, Publishers, Inc. All rights reserved. Printed in the United States of America. No part of this book may be used or reproduced in any manner whatsoever without written permission except in the case of brief quotations embodied in critical articles and reviews. For information address Harper & Row, Publishers, Inc., 10 East 53rd Street, New York, NY 10022. Published simultaneously in Canada by Fitzhenry & Whiteside Limited, Toronto.

FIRST EDITION

Designed by Alma Orenstein

Library of Congress Cataloging-in-Publication Data

Wallach, Leah, 1947–
    Food values—calcium.

    1. Food—Calcium content—Tables. 2. Calcium in the body. I. Title.
TX553.C23W35 1989   641.1'7   88-45547
ISBN 0-06-096221-6

89 90 91 92 93 AG/BC 10 9 8 7 6 5 4 3 2 1

Contents

Acknowledgments

I'd like to thank Laura Hickey, Shawn Connor, and Tim Bishop who assisted me in the rather tedious task of entering data, and Alex Cantor who typed and helped organize my correspondence with the food processors. I'd like also to acknowledge Helene A. Guthrie, whom I have never met, but whose textbook, *Introductory Nutrition,* proved a most useful reference during the early stages of this project.

I'm especially grateful to the scientists who allowed me to consult with them in the course of this book, and particularly to Dr. B. Lawrence Riggs of the Mayo Clinic; Dr. Christopher Cann of the University of California at San Francisco; Dr. Brian Morgan of the Institute of Human Nutrition, Columbia University; Dr. Van S. Hubbard of the National Institute of Arthritis, Diabetes, Digestive, and Kidney Diseases; Dr. Leon Ellenbogen of Lederly Pharmaceuticals; Dr. Robert Recker of Creighton University; Dr. Harold Schedl of University Hospital, Iowa City; Dr. David McCarron of Oregon Health Sciences University; Dr. Martin Lipkin of Memorial Sloan-Kettering Cancer Center; Dr. Edward Frohlich, Distinguished Scientist and Vice President for Academic Affairs, Alton Ochsner Medical Foundation; and Dr. Dennis Ponton, chairman of the Nutrition and Food Science Department, Buffalo State College.

Introduction

There was a poster of the four major food groups on the wall of my elementary-school classroom and of thousands of classrooms like it. "Dairy" was represented by a picture of a glass of milk and a wedge of cheese on a plate. An arrow led to the caption: "Calcium for strong bones and teeth."

Most of us who grew up with that poster grew up taking calcium for granted. We stopped drinking milk with our meals as we got older and cut back on cheese when we were worried about weight control with no fear of dire consequences. Then, in the 1980s, calcium suddenly became a celebrity nutrient, written up in newspapers, discussed on the nightly news, even featured in *People* magazine. Calcium owes its rising reputation to the growing awareness that between 15 and 24 million Americans over the age of 45, mostly women, have a condition called osteoporosis: their bones are normal, but the quantity of their bone mass has diminished, making them susceptible to fractures. Osteoporosis is responsible for about 1.3 million fractures each year, most of them in the vertebrae, hip, or forearm, and 12% to 20% of the people who fracture a hip die as a result of complications. Since calcium builds strong bones and teeth, researchers began investigating the relationship of calcium intake to osteoporosis. Initial work suggested that low calcium intake increased the risk of fractures, and soon higher calcium intake was being touted as a way of preventing osteoporosis.

The virtues of calcium, it quickly turned out, had been oversold. Further research has made it clear that increased calcium intake alone will not prevent bone loss. On the other hand, a considerable body of research suggests that many Americans, especially women, would be healthier if throughout their lives they consumed more calcium than they do now. Most American women at present get between 475 and 575 milligrams of calcium a day from their diet, considerably less than the RDA, or daily allowance for adults recommended by the Food and Nutrition Board of the National Research Council. The RDA of calcium is 800 milligrams—and some doctors think the RDA should be raised for women.

The current RDAs for calcium by age are:

	Years	Milligrams of Calcium
Infants	birth to 6 months	360
	6 months to 1 year	540
Children of either sex	1–10	800
Adults of either sex	11–18	1,200
	over 18	800
Pregnant and lactating women		400 above recommended daily allowance for woman's age group

Calcium in the Body

Calcium compounds are the most abundant minerals in the human body, accounting for between 1½% and 2% of our total weight.

Adult teeth contain about 1% of the body's calcium. This calcium, which is a major component of tooth enamel and of the inner layer of the tooth, called dentin, is deposited during childhood, while the teeth are still in the gums. None is added after the teeth erupt; the dentin and the enamel you have now are all you will ever have.

About 98% of the calcium in the body is in the bones. There are two kinds of bone. Cortical bone looks smooth and solid. Trabecular bone has a spongy, honeycomb structure. Every bone in the body contains some of each type, but some bones, like the long bones of the arms and legs, are mostly cortical, while other kinds of bones, like the vertebrae of the spine, have a higher proportion of trabecular bone.

Bone is a complex living tissue supplied with nerves, nourished by blood, and bathed in fluid. Like most living tissues, it is constantly being broken down, or resorbed, and reformed, a process called bone remodeling.

From birth until early adulthood, the body produces more new bone tissue than it loses through breakdown. Trabecular bone formation is completed in the early 20s, cortical bone formation in the mid- or late 30s. Bone remodeling does not stop, however. Bones continue to be broken down and reshaped throughout the lifespan. But as adults age, the rate of bone breakdown begins to exceed the rate of bone formation. The rate of bone loss is more rapid among women than among men, but it is slow in both sexes at first. Then, at menopause, women's rate of bone loss accelerates suddenly and remains highly elevated for five or six years. As women move into their 60s, their rate of bone loss slows again and begins to approximate that of men.

About 1% of the body's calcium, the calcium that isn't in the bones and teeth, is distributed in the body and the blood, where it helps maintain cell membranes, aids muscle contractions and nerve impulse conduction, regulates heartbeat and cellular growth, stimulates blood clotting, and facilitates the absorption of vitamin B_{12}, the activation of various enzymes, the secretion of insulin, and the response of the cells to certain neurotransmitters and hormones. We can't do without it. The circulation of calcium to the cells through the blood is so important to our survival that the body does not allow calcium blood levels to go up or down by more than 3%. When there is not enough calcium in the blood, calcium is withdrawn from the bones to make up the difference. In fact, one of the functions of bone is to serve as a storehouse for calcium so that proper blood levels can be maintained.

Calcium Metabolism

Some of the calcium in the bones is dissolved to keep the supply of calcium in the blood constant, and some of the calcium absorbed from food is used to rebuild bone. Several feedback systems work together to regulate this process and keep blood calcium levels stable. When levels of calcium in the blood fall, the parathyroid gland secretes a hormone that signals the kidneys to excrete less calcium and accelerates the release of exchangeable bone calcium into the blood. The hormone also stimulates the liver and kidneys to convert vitamin D to its active form. The vitamin D derivative increases the absorption of calcium in the small intestine, helps the parathyroid hormone release bone calcium, and further increases calcium retention by the kidneys. When blood levels of calcium return to normal, the secretion of parathyroid hormone goes down.

A different hormone, calcitonin, is secreted when calcium blood levels become too high. Calcitonin inhibits the breakdown of bone. When calcium blood levels or dietary intake of calcium is high, the body also activates less vitamin D. That means calcium absorption is more efficient when intake is low. For this reason, increasing calcium in the diet doesn't lead to a proportional increase in the amount of calcium absorbed by the body. It does lead to an absolute increase, however.

Many other substances have a role in calcium metabolism, a complicated process that is not fully understood. Exercise also appears to influence bone remodeling. Inactivity is bad for the skeleton, and weight-bearing exercise like jogging, tennis, aerobics, and walking may help maintain bone mass. Vigorous weight-bearing exercise, however, especially in older people whose bones are already weakened, is as likely to cause fractures as to prevent them.

Osteoporosis

Researchers don't fully understand the genesis of osteoporosis. It's thought to result from multiple causes, and to develop for different reasons in different people. But researchers have been able to identify a number of risk factors for the disease. A risk factor is a trait or habit that is more common among people with a disease than among people without it. A risk factor is not a cause. Some people with many risk factors for osteoporosis do not get fractures, and some people with osteoporosis have no risk factors for it.

Sex and age are two important risk factors. Rates of osteoporosis are much higher among women than among men. All women lose bone rapidly in the years immediately following menopause, and a subgroup of women (not all) lose bone, particularly trabecular bone, at an especially high rate. Fifteen to twenty years after menopause, they may develop Type I osteoporosis, which is characterized by painful and deforming fractures of the vertebrae and forearms.

Osteoporosis is a disease of people over 45. Menopause occurs in most women in middle age, and Type I osteoporosis doesn't develop until some years later. Another type of osteoporosis, Type II, characterized by hip and vertebral fractures, afflicts both men and women over 70 but is more common among women. Women are more prone to the disorder partly because they lose bone rapidly at menopause and consequently enter old age with their bone mass already diminished, and partly because they have less bone in the first place. People who start life with large, strong skeletons can afford to lose more of their bone mass before they will be prone to fractures.

How much bone a person has at the beginning of adult life is at least partly a matter of heredity. On the average, women begin adulthood with 30% less bone than men, and small, thin women are at greater risk of osteoporosis than large women. Other hereditary factors may play a role in osteoporosis, which tends to run in families. Some researchers believe that a chemical imbalance in bone metabolism may be involved.

Additional risk factors include smoking, alcoholism, and heavy caffeine consumption (more than 4 or 5 cups of coffee a day). Certain illnesses, medical procedures, and medications also increase the risk of developing the disease. Insufficient dietary intake of calcium may be another risk factor, but just how important a factor is the subject of much debate.

Researchers have generally found that higher dietary intake of calcium is associated with fewer fractures. But such studies do not prove that low calcium intake causes people to lose bone mass, only that they are associated. (Cause and association are very different: for example, more young people than old people get head injuries in motorcycle accidents—but being young is not a cause of head injury in motorcycle accidents.)

To see if calcium intake could prevent rapid bone loss at menopause, a number of scientists undertook intervention studies: they asked a group of menopausal women to increase their calcium intake (generally in the form of supplements) and compared them with a similar group of untreated women. The results of these studies were quite consistent: the women who consumed more calcium lost bone just as rapidly as the untreated women. Estrogen replacement therapy, on the other hand, very effectively retarded bone loss. The researchers concluded that it is not lack of calcium itself, but inability to use available calcium to reform bone at an adequate rate because of hormonal changes, that is responsible for the loss of skeletal mass at menopause. The researchers did find that calcium can play a useful role as an adjunct to estrogen replacement therapy. If women have a high intake of calcium, the amount of estrogen they need to prevent bone loss can be significantly reduced. Reducing the dose of estrogen probably reduces the risk of side effects.

As a result of these recent studies, calcium intake among the middle aged is not considered as important a factor in the genesis of osteoporosis as it was a few years ago. Researchers still believe, however, that adequate calcium consumption throughout the lifespan is important. They are increasingly emphasizing the need for teenage girls to get enough of the mineral. Many doctors are now inclined to think that the statistical association between high calcium intake and lower incidence of osteoporosis found in many studies indicates that women with more calcium in their diet developed bigger, stronger skeletons when they were young and their bones were still growing. Consequently, doctors are urging young women to meet the RDA of 1,200 milligrams for years 11 to 18 to ensure that they develop the strongest bones possible within the limits of their genetic potential.

The RDA for Calcium—Is It Enough?

There is some controversy about just how much dietary calcium constitutes optimal consumption. Most researchers believe that there is a threshold below which there is a relationship between calcium intake and bone mass and above which further intake of calcium has little or no effect. The threshold is probably different for different people and for the same person at different stages of life. Doctors who recommend that the RDA for adult women be increased argue that calcium balance studies are the best available technique for estimating this threshold.

Calcium balance studies compare the amount of calcium in the food a person eats with the amount excreted in urine or feces. Calcium equilibrium exists when a person is neither storing calcium nor losing it. Many researchers who have conducted calcium balance studies would like to see the RDA for adult women raised from 800 to 1,000 milligrams. Some also recommend that elderly women increase their intake to 1,200 or 1,500 milligrams on the premise (as yet unproved) that increased intake of calcium might compensate for the decreased absorption of the mineral that often accompanies old age.

A respectable minority argues that the RDA for calcium should not be raised (a few people even argue that it should be lowered). They make the following points:

- The results of calcium balance studies are not consistent, and short-term and longer-term studies yield different results.
- There is no illness that can be classified as calcium deficiency, no hard evidence that Americans suffer any ill effects because of low calcium intake, and no hard evidence that increasing calcium intake could prevent or retard osteoporosis.
- There is evidence that the body adjusts to lower intake of dietary calcium by absorbing more of it.
- Increased calcium intake after age 35 obviously does not lead to increased bone formation, since no one over 35 grows a bigger skeleton no matter how much calcium he or she consumes.

- Meeting a 1,000-milligram requirement within a balanced diet and without increasing caloric intake would be difficult for the average American woman and would involve very careful meal planning.

New RDAs for all nutrients, representing consensus opinions, may soon be released. Meanwhile the average American woman needn't worry unduly about the controversy. Nutrients aren't drugs, where it's important to get an exact dosage. If you find that you're among the many American women who get less than 600 milligrams of calcium a day from their food, you would be wise to alter your eating habits to get more. You might decide to aim for an intake of 800 or 1,000 milligrams—but there is no need to be rigorous. If you end up consuming 700 milligrams of calcium one day, 1,100 the next, and 850 the third, most doctors would agree you're eating well.

Calcium Toxicity

There is no evidence of harmful effects from calcium intake of up to 2,000 milligrams (2 grams) per day. Doctors generally suggest that people limit intake to a maximum of 1,500 milligrams per day. If a person's diet is well balanced and nutritionally sound, intake up to this level will not affect absorption of other minerals, elevate blood calcium levels, or cause deposits in soft tissues or kidney damage. There is an exception: dietary calcium stimulates kidney-stone formation in some, though not all, patients with kidney stones. People with kidney stones or a family history of kidney stones should not increase their calcium intake without consulting a doctor.

Calcium Intake, High Blood Pressure, and Colon Cancer

Several studies have found that higher intakes of dietary calcium are associated with lower incidence of hypertension (high blood pressure). Preliminary research at Memorial Sloan-Kettering Cancer Center also suggests that increased calcium intake can lower the risk of developing colon cancer among people thought to be susceptible to that disease. The majority of doctors feels that more research is needed before any claims can be made about the relationship between calcium intake and either high blood pressure or colon cancer. Meanwhile, both the doctors who are enthusiastic about these lines of research and the National Institutes of Health recommend simply that people meet the calcium RDA.

Calcium, Other Nutrients, and Bone Health

A number of other nutrients affect or at one time or another have been thought to affect the body's ability to use calcium and to remodel bone.

Vitamin D We need 300 to 440 International Units of vitamin D in order to absorb calcium from food efficiently. However, since vitamin D also helps the body withdraw calcium from the bones, high levels can contribute to bone loss. High levels are also toxic.

Vitamin D is produced by the skin when it has contact with sunlight. It is found in fortified milk, fish liver oil, and in small quantities in some other foods. Vitamin D deficiency is rare in America except among the homebound and among those elderly who aren't able to metabolize the vitamin well. Excessive intake is uncommon also. The skin regulates the amount of the chemical it makes, so you can't get an overdose from sunbathing, and it's hard to get too much vitamin D from food. You can consume dangerous amounts if you use supplements.

Lactose Lactose, a sugar found abundantly in milk, improves the absorption of calcium by infants and is thought to aid in calcium absorption by adults as well.

Fat Milk fat does not aid in the absorption of calcium from dairy products. Skim and nonfat dry milk contain slightly more calcium than regular milk, and the calcium in the low-fat products may also be easier to absorb.

Protein Protein consumption increases the excretion of calcium in the urine. However, American diets high in protein also tend to be high in calcium, which one study suggests may compensate for the slight increase in calcium loss.

Plant Foods Though there is little hard data on the subject, most nutritionists believe that the calcium in vegetables and grains is not very well absorbed by the human body. Three substances found in plant foods decrease calcium absorption: oxalic acid, phytic acid, and fiber. Oxalic acid combines with calcium to form calcium oxalate, which the body cannot digest. Some vegetables that are very rich in calcium, including beet greens, Swiss chard, sorrel, and spinach, are also high in oxalic acid, which means that much of the calcium they contain may not be available to the body. Phytic acid, found in the outer husks of cereals (in bran, oatmeal, and whole grains), also binds calcium. Finally, fiber, which is supplied by plant foods, is believed to decrease slightly the absorption of minerals, though the body has some ability to adjust to a high-fiber diet.

Vitamin A Megadoses of vitamin A may stimulate bone loss. A woman needs only 800 retinol equivalents (4,000 International Units) a day; a man 1,000 retinol equivalents (5,000 International Units).

Phosphorus Both calcium and phosphorus are needed to build bone. Many nutritionists believe that both minerals are utilized best when consumed in the right proportions— but disagree about what the proportions should be.

The typical American diet contains considerably more phosphorus than calcium because of our high consumption of protein-rich foods, carbonated beverages, and foods preserved with phosphorus compounds. Very high intake of phosphorus has been shown to lead to calcium loss in animals, and as a result, nutritionists used to urge people to reduce phosphorus intake. However, studies of human beings have not found any relationship between phosphorus intake and calcium utilization at the levels involved in a normal diet, and there is generally less concern about phosphorus intake than there was a few years ago.

Magnesium Some researchers have been concerned about possible interactions between calcium and magnesium, and have suggested that people increase magnesium intake as they increase calcium intake to maintain a balance of one part magnesium to two parts calcium. There is, however, no evidence suggesting that increased magnesium intake will facilitate calcium absorption or that increased calcium intake will create magnesium deficiencies, provided that magnesium is already present in the diet at adequate levels.

Dietary Sources of Calcium

Three-quarters of the calcium in the American diet comes from milk and milk products, which are the best sources of the mineral. Dairy products contain more calcium per serving than any other group of foods. The calcium they contain is well absorbed by the body, and they are widely available and relatively low in cost, can be consumed in many different forms, and contain many nutrients in addition to calcium. The easiest way to increase calcium intake is to eat more dairy products.

A cup of milk—skim, low-fat, or regular—contains between 250 and 300 milligrams of calcium. Yogurt contains slightly more calcium and calories per cup. Cheeses vary quite a bit in calcium content. Cottage cheese contains less calcium per serving than most hard cheeses, because some of the calcium in the milk from which it is made is removed in the preparation process. Cream cheese is also a relatively poor source of calcium, because it is mostly fat. Dairy desserts like ice milk, ice cream, and custard provide significant amounts of calcium.

About 30 million Americans get gas and stomach cramps when they drink milk, because they don't produce enough lactase, the enzyme that digests the milk sugar lactose. The problem becomes more common as people age, and is more common among people of African and Asian ancestry than among people of European ancestry. Most lactase-deficient adults can still enjoy some dairy foods. Some can handle milk in small quantities or can eat hard cheese, which may contain less lactose per serving than milk. Many can eat yogurt, which contains an enzyme that helps absorb lactose. Drugstores sell Lact-Aid, an enzyme preparation that can be added to a quart of milk to predigest the lactose, and cartons of Lact-Aid milk are sold commercially in many supermarkets.

Good nondairy sources of calcium include canned sardines and salmon eaten with the bones, cooked dried peas, fortified (not regular) soy milk, broccoli, and dark green leafy vegetables like turnip greens that do not contain oxalic acid. Soybean curd or tofu is an especially good source of calcium. Most tofu is prepared with a sea-salt preparation called nigari and contains about 130 milligrams of calcium per ½ cup regular or 250 milligrams per ½ cup firm. Tofu prepared with calcium sulfate contains a whopping 435 milligrams of calcium per ½ cup regular or 860 milligrams per ½ cup firm.

Foods that contain between 20 and 50 milligrams of calcium per serving are not considered good sources of calcium in themselves, but several of these foods eaten together in the course of the day can contribute a significant amount of calcium to the diet. Most people will find it difficult, however, to take in 800 or 1,000 milligrams without eating dairy products or some of the other calcium-rich foods mentioned above.

Calcium, Fat, Cholesterol, and Weight Gain

If you raise your intake of calcium simply by adding calcium-rich foods to your diet, you will gain weight. To maintain your present weight, you have to substitute calcium-rich foods for foods with the same number of calories.

The National Institutes of Health and the American Heart Association both recommend that Americans reduce the number of calories in their diet supplied by fat to 30% from the present average of 37% and limit cholesterol intake to a maximum of 300 milligrams. You can include dairy products in your diet and still stay within these limits. Dairy products contain less cholesterol per serving than meat, poultry, and shellfish. A cup of nonfat (not low-fat) yogurt contains virtually no cholesterol; a cup of skim milk, 5 milligrams. Regular milk and hard cheese contain between 25 and 34 milligrams per serving. You can have three or four servings of these foods and still have a large hunk of your cholesterol budget left over.

From 40% to 50% of the calories in whole milk and over 70% of the calories in hard cheese come from fat, but fat supplies less than 30% of the calories in buttermilk, low-fat milk, and low-fat yogurt. Skim and nonfat milk and milk products contain only a trace of fat. Ice milk contains less fat than ice cream, and among some ice creams, the cheaper brands are less rich. You can, of course, eat some of the higher-fat dairy products if you like them, provided you cut back on fat in the rest of your diet to compensate.

The National Institutes of Health also recommend that only one-third of the calories from fat come from saturated fat. A little over half the fat in dairy products is saturated, so you may want to compensate for dairy fat intake by preparing foods with fats and oils that are primarily monosaturated or polyunsaturated.

Supplements

Supplements are an easy way for the lactose intolerant and people who don't like dairy foods to get additional calcium. Supplements have no calories and contain no fats or cholesterol—they're just hunks of mineral.

Almost all nutritionists believe it's best to get our nutrients from foods, not pills. It's not hard to consume excessive quantities of a nutrient by using single nutrient supplements; it's very hard to do so through diet alone. Some nutritionists also believe that calcium supplementation, even at modest levels, is more likely to lead to imbalances than is dietary calcium, because the supplements contain only calcium while foods provide several nutrients at once. On the other hand, numerous studies of the relationship between calcium intake and osteoporosis and other conditions have been conducted using supplements that appear to be both safe and effective.

Calcium isn't stable alone; it has to be combined with another element. To make supplements, calcium is most commonly combined with carbonate, lactate, gluconate, citrate, or phosphate. The tablets are bulky, and only a portion of the bulk consists of calcium. If you decide to use a supplement, read the label to see how much calcium each tablet contains so you can figure out how many you will need to take.

The supplement most commonly recommended is calcium carbonate, which contains the highest percentage of calcium and is relatively inexpensive. It can, however, cause constipation in some people.

Some antacids contain calcium carbonate. A Tums tablet, for example, contains about 200 milligrams of calcium carbonate and 3 calories and is cheap. Taking a small number of antacid tablets over the course of the day will not upset your stomach, but taking eight or more at once may, paradoxically, stimulate stomach acid secretions. Before using any antacid as a supplement, look on the label and make sure it contains calcium, not aluminum.

Experts disagree about the best way to take supplements. Most recommend taking them with meals, not on an empty stomach.

Another way to take supplements is to eat fortified foods. Nutritionists point out, however, that the calcium in fortified foods may not be absorbed well, or may be effective in one kind of food and not another. Calcium-fortified orange juice has been tested, and the calcium it contains is well absorbed.

If you decide to take supplements, don't take excessive quantities. You can use this book to calculate how much calcium you are currently getting from your diet. You should use supplements only to make up the difference between your dietary intake of calcium and the amount you would like to consume. For example, if your daily intake from food is 500 milligrams and you want to raise your intake to 800 milligrams, don't take an 800-milligram supplement—300 milligrams is sufficient.

How to Use This Book

Food Values: Calcium provides the number of milligrams of calcium, the number of grams of fat, and the number of calories in thousands of foods.

The foods are divided into forty-eight categories covering all the things we eat and drink. As you flip through the pages of this book you'll quickly see where various foods are located. If you can't find a food in the category where you think it belongs, check the head note at the beginning of the category or refer to the table of contents. When products could be classified in more than one category, we have tried to include a "see also" reference.

Each category begins with an alphabetical listing of generic food items, with fresh products listed before processed foods; for instance, you'll find fresh peaches before canned peaches. Following the generic foods are all brand-name products alphabetized by the name that is most easily recognized, either the name of the manufacturing company, of the product line, or of the product itself. For instance, Campbell's soups are listed under Campbell, the company name, while Ortega sauces are listed under Ortega, the product line name, rather than under the manufacturer, Nabisco, and Kit Kat candy bar is listed under Kit Kat, because it is better known by its product name than by the fact that it is a Hershey product. Under each brand name, specific products are generally listed alphabetically; Aunt Jemima French toast, for example, precedes Aunt Jemima pancakes. We found, however, as most alphabetizers do, that some items could be listed in more than one way; we had to make choices. Under Fleischmann's margarine, for instance, diet follows regular though it begins with *d*, and, in the legumes category, split peas are under *s* not *p*. If you don't find a food under the first letter of the first word of its name, try looking for it under the first letter of another word in the name. The cross-references should help here too.

Be sure to look for foods in the form in which you eat them: the way foods are prepared changes their nutrient values. A cup of cooked turnip greens, for example, contains more calcium than a cup of raw greens, because there is more vegetable and less water in the cooked product. A soup prepared with milk contains more calcium, fat, and calories than the same food prepared with water. Foods prepared with whole milk contain more fat and calories than the same foods prepared with skim milk.

We've used the portion sizes that Americans use—cups, ounces, or serving units—and when available, we've used two kinds of measures; for example, "3 cookies = 1 oz." Serving units are the easiest portions to measure; it's easier to count cookies than to weigh them. However, you can compare only serving units of the same weight. For example, if a package of Brand X frozen lasagna weighs 10 ounces, and a package of Brand Y frozen lasagna weighs 18 ounces, the calorie, fat, and calcium values will probably all be higher for Brand Y than for Brand X, because the portion size is bigger. But Brand Y might contain fewer calories and less fat and calcium per ounce than Brand X. To compare two products of different sizes, divide the values for each product by the number of ounces it contains and then compare the values for 1 ounce.

Please note the difference between weight measures and volume measures. Measuring cups measure fluid ounces. An ounce of water by weight fills a measuring cup to the 1-ounce line. But volume and weight are very different kinds of measures for solid foods. An ounce of unpopped popcorn, which is dense, wouldn't fill a measuring cup, for example, but an ounce of popped popcorn, which is airy, would fill more than one. In this book, portions for solid food given in ounces refer to weight. Fluid ounces (fl oz), cups (c), teaspoons (t), and tablespoons (T) refer to volume measurements. Since we don't ordinarily weigh our food, we've given volume and weight measurements when both are available and useful. For example, we've indicated how much of a measuring cup would be filled by an ounce of a given cold cereal when this information was available.

All the values given here are approximations. No two apples, chicken breasts, or rolls are exactly alike. Data represent averages for several samples.

Figures provided by different sources may not be exactly comparable. The U.S. Department of Agriculture (USDA) and various manufacturers may use different analytical procedures to analyze nutrient content and may round off the data in different ways. In the USDA *Composition of Food* series, our source of information about generic and fresh food, values are given to hundredths or thousandths. We rounded off the figures to the nearest whole unit. For example, we list 68.4 calories as 68 calories and 68½ calories as 69 calories. When an item contained less than ½ calorie, less than ½ gram of fat, or less than ½ milligram of calcium, we listed the value as a "trace" (tr) (1 gram equals .035 ounce; 1 milligram is one-thousandth of a gram).

Many manufacturers use a simpler rounding off system, approved by the Food and Drug Administration (FDA), which regulates food labels. Calories between 0 and 20 may be given in increments of 2; between 20 and 50 in increments of 5; and above 50 in increments of 5 or 10. This means that there's no point in counting single calories when comparing products; a product listed as containing 107 calories, another listed as containing 105, and a third listed as containing 110 may actually contain the same amount of food energy.

To facilitate nutrient labeling on food products, the FDA has condensed the Recommended Daily Allowances of the Food and Nutrition Board to form a simpler system of recommended daily requirements called the USRDAs. The USRDA of calcium for adults is 1,000 milligrams. Information about the calcium content of processed foods was sometimes given to us, as it is also given on labels, in terms of the percentage of the USRDA contained in a portion of the product. If the percentage is less than 2, for example, it is usually just listed as "less than 2%." If the percentage is between 2 and 10, it is rounded in 2% increments; between 10 and 50, in 5% increments; and over 50, in 10% increments. When manufacturers provided us with calcium values in this form, we converted the percentage of the USRDA (the percentage of 1,000 milligrams) to the number of milligrams by multiplying the percentage by 10 (for example, 15% of 1,000 milligrams is 150 milligrams). When percentages over 50% were rounded to the nearest 10, this system yielded only very approximate values for calcium content. If a brand-name product contained 60% of the USRDA of calcium, for example, we listed 600 milligrams; the product might actually provide anywhere between 560 and 640 milligrams of the mineral.

When information about the calcium or fat content of a food was not available, we put a question mark in the appropriate column.

This book represents the best information now available. Since food manufacturers constantly change recipes and product sizes and develop new products, some information contained here may be quickly outdated.

Calculating the Amount of Calcium and Fat in Your Diet

To get an idea of the number of milligrams of calcium, grams of fat, and calories in your present diet, keep a complete record of everything (every mouthful) you eat and drink for three days, including one weekend day. Right after you finish a meal or snack or beverage, write down what you ate, how it was prepared, and the portion by volume (cups, teaspoons), weight (ounces), units (1 medium apple, 1 English muffin), or all three. To get a feeling for different food sizes, measure your food when you are at home. For example, put the cereal in a measuring cup before you put it into a bowl to see how much you use, then pour milk into a measuring cup before you pour it over the cereal. You may find that the portion sizes used in this book are smaller than the ones you use. For example, for many American adults, a typical main course portion of spaghetti is 2 cups, not the 1 cup listed as a portion here.

At the end of the three days, look up the calcium, fat, and calorie values for all the foods you have eaten, add them together, and divide by three to figure your average daily intake. If your average daily intake of calcium is less than 800 or 1,000 milligrams, whichever level of intake you decide to make your goal, you can use the book to find ways to make up the difference. First look up some high-calcium foods, like dairy products, tofu, or sardines. Find some items you like, and try to substitute them for items in your present diet that contain little calcium but about the same amount of fat and calories. You might also look up your favorite foods to see if you can increase your calcium intake by preparing them in a different way or choosing a different brand.

You can also use the listings to calculate the percentage of calories in your diet that is provided by fats, and to reduce the fat in your diet, if necessary, at the same time that you increase your calcium intake.

Fat holds energy in very concentrated form; each gram of fat contains about 9 calories, compared to 4 calories for a gram of protein or carbohydrate. To figure the percentage of calories supplied by fat in a given food, multiply the number of grams of fat by 9 to get the number of calories supplied by fat, then divide by the total number of calories. For example, an egg contains 6 grams of fat, which provide 6 times 9, or 54, calories. The total number of calories in an egg is 79. The percentage of those calories provided by fat is 54/79, or 68%.

One way to increase calcium intake while keeping fat intake down is simply to choose skim or part-skim dairy products and other high-calcium foods that are low in fat. This could lead to a very unsatisfying diet, however. It makes more sense to look at the percentage of calories you are getting from fat in whole meals or whole days. You'll see that there is room in a healthful diet for some high-fat foods. For example, while 70% of the calories in Swiss cheese eaten alone come from fat, less than a third of the calories provided by a meal of a cup of chicken noodle soup, 1 ounce of Swiss cheese, a slice of tomato, two slices of dry rye toast, and an apple come from fat. Ice cream is a high-fat food, but if it adds joy to your life you can enjoy some— if you reduce the amount of fat in one of your other meals to compensate.

Enjoying food is important: it's part of enjoying life, which is good for your health. We hope this book will help you plan meals that are as pleasurable as they are nutritious.

Sources

1. *Food Values of Portions Commonly Used, 14th Edition*, Jean A. T. Pennington and Helen Nichols Church, Harper & Row, 1985.
2. *Nutritive Value of Foods*, U.S. Department of Agriculture, Nutrition Information Service, Home and Garden Bulletin #72, revised 1981.
3. *Composition of Food Series*, U.S. Department of Agriculture, Science and Education Administration:

    8-1 *Dairy and Egg Products*, revised November 1976.

    8-3 *Baby Foods*, revised December 1978.

    8-4 *Fats and Oils*, revised June 1979.

    8-5 *Poultry Products*, revised August 1979.

    8-6 *Soups, Sauces and Gravies*, revised February 1980.

    8-7 *Sausages and Luncheon Meats*, revised September 1980.

    8-8 *Breakfast Cereals*, revised July 1982.

    8-9 *Fruits and Fruit Juices*, revised August 1982.

    8-10 *Pork Products*, revised August 1983.

    8-11 *Vegetables and Vegetable Products*, revised August 1984.

    8-12 *Nut and Seed Products*, revised September 1984.

    8-13 *Beef Products*, revised August 1986.

    8-14 *Beverages*, revised May 1986.

    8-15 *Finfish and Shellfish Products*, revised September 1987.

    8-16 *Legumes and Legume Products*, revised December 1986.

Information about brand-name products was supplied by the food processing companies themselves or taken from the above sources.

Abbreviations

c	=	cup
cal	=	calories
chol	=	cholesterol
diam	=	diameter
g	=	grams
lb	=	pounds
mg	=	milligrams
oz	=	ounces
pkg	=	package
pkt	=	packet
sat fat	=	saturated fat
T	=	tablespoon
t	=	teaspoon
tr	=	trace
w/	=	with
w/out	=	without
?	=	not available, or not known at this time
<	=	less than
≤	=	less than or equal to

FOOD VALUES

Calcium

	Portion	Calcium (mg)	Total Fat (g)	Total Calor
❑ **ALCOHOLIC BEVERAGES** *See* BEVERAGES				
❑ **BABY FOOD** *See* INFANT & TODDLER FOODS				
❑ **BAKING INGREDIENTS**				
baking powder, sodium aluminum sulfate				
w/monocalcium phosphate monohydrate	1 t	58	0	5
w/monocalcium phosphate monohydrate, calcium sulfate	1 t	183	0	5
straight phosphate	1 t	239	0	5
low-sodium	1 t	207	0	5
candied fruit				
apricot	1 medium	4	tr	101
cherry	3 large	?	tr	51
maraschino cherry	2 medium	?	tr	19
citron	1 oz	24	tr	89
fig	1 piece	20	tr	90
ginger root	1 oz	?	tr	95
peel of grapefruit/lemon/ orange	1 oz	?	tr	89
pear	1 oz	?	tr	85
pineapple	1 slice	12	tr	120
cornmeal *See* FLOURS & CORNMEALS				
cornstarch *See* FLOURS & CORNMEALS				
flour *See* FLOURS & CORNMEALS				
pastry puff dough	1 oz	3	10	129
patty shell	2½ oz	0	19	240
piecrust				
crumb	5.8 oz	113	64	866
from mix w/vegetable shortening	for 2-crust 9″ pie	131	93	1,485
frozen	1/16 crust = 1 oz	3	8	130
graham cracker	4.8 oz	8	10	159
homemade, w/vegetable shortening	for 9″ pie	25	60	900
yeast				
baker's, dry, active	1 pkg	3	tr	20
brewer's, dry	1 T	17	tr	25
torula	1 T	42	tr	28

	Portion	Calcium (mg)	Total Fat (g)	Total Calor
■ BRAND NAME				
Baker's				
COCONUT				
Angel Flake, bag	⅓ c	<20	8	120
CHOCOLATE				
German's sweet chocolate	1 oz	<20	10	140
semisweet chocolate	1 oz	<20	9	140
semisweet chocolate–flavored chips	¼ c	60	9	190
semisweet real chocolate chips	¼ c	<20	12	200
unsweetened chocolate	1 oz	20	15	140
Davis				
baking powder	1 t	60	0	8
Hershey				
milk chocolate chips	1 oz	40	8	150
semisweet chocolate chips, regular & miniature	¼ c or 1½ oz	<20	12	220
unsweetened baking chocolate	1 oz	20	16	190
Nabisco				
graham cracker crumbs	2 T	<20	1	60
Reese's				
peanut butter–flavored chips	¼ c or 1½ oz	60	13	230
Sunshine				
graham cracker crumbs	1 c	80	14	550

❏ BAKING MIXES

cakes & pastries, prepared from mix *See* DESSERTS: CAKES, PASTRIES, & PIES
pancakes, prepared from mix *See* BREAKFAST FOODS, PREPARED
pie fillings, prepared from mix *See* DESSERTS: CUSTARDS, GELATINS, PUDDINGS, & PIE FILLINGS
waffles, prepared from mix *See* BREAKFAST FOODS, PREPARED

■ BRAND NAME

Arrowhead Mills				
biscuit mix	2 oz	150	1	100
bran muffin mix	2 muffins	80	7	270
corn bread mix	1 oz	100	1	100

	Portion	Calcium (mg)	Total Fat (g)	Total Calor
Aunt Jemima				
Easy Mix coffee cake	1.3 oz	58	4	162
Easy Mix corn bread	1.7 oz	15	6	205
Dromedary				
corn bread, prepared	2″×2″ piece	60	3	130
corn muffin, prepared	1 muffin	40	4	120
gingerbread, prepared	2″×2″ piece	20	2	100
pound cake, prepared	½″ slice	20	6	150
Fearn				
BAKING MIXES				
brown rice	½ c	350	3	215
rice	½ c	400	1	260
whole-wheat	½ c	250	2	210
BREAD & MUFFIN MIXES				
bran muffin	1½ oz	6	1	110
corn bread	⅓ c dry	40	2	160
CAKE MIXES				
banana	⅓ c dry	60	2	130
carob	⅓ c dry	80	2	120
carrot	⅓ c dry	60	2	140
spice	⅓ c dry	60	3	140
Flako				
corn muffin mix	1 oz	18	2	116
pie crust mix	1.7 oz	48	14	244
popover mix	1 oz	9	1	102
Jell-O				
cheesecake, prepared w/ whole milk	⅛ of 8″ cake	150	13	280
chocolate mousse pie, prepared w/whole milk	⅛ pie	80	15	250
coconut cream pie, prepared w/whole milk	⅛ pie	60	17	260
Pillsbury				
All Ready pie crust	⅛ of 2-crust pie	0	15	240
biscuits, bread, rolls *See* BREADS, ROLLS, BISCUITS, & MUFFINS				
Royal				
chocolate mint pie mix	⅛ pie	40	15	260
chocolate mousse pie mix	⅛ pie	40	12	230
lemon meringue pie mix	⅛ pie	20	11	310
lite cheese cake mix	⅛ pie	60	10	210
Real cheese cake mix	⅛ pie	<20	9	280

❏ **BEANS** *See* LEGUMES & LEGUME PRODUCTS

	Portion	Calcium (mg)	Total Fat (g)	Total Calor

❑ BEEF, FRESH & CURED
See also PROCESSED MEAT & POULTRY PRODUCTS

NOTE: "1 lb raw" refers to the edible portion of meat yielded when 1 pound of the raw product is cooked.

Beef, Fresh

BRISKET

Lean & Fat

	Portion	Calcium (mg)	Total Fat (g)	Total Calor
whole, all grades, braised	3 oz cooked	7	28	332
	1 lb raw	28	104	1,258
flat half, all grades, braised	3 oz cooked	8	30	347
	1 lb raw	29	112	1,311
point half, all grades, braised	3 oz cooked	7	25	311
	1 lb raw	26	93	1,172

Lean Only

	Portion	Calcium (mg)	Total Fat (g)	Total Calor
whole, all grades, braised	3 oz cooked	5	11	205
	1 lb raw	12	27	513
flat half, all grades, braised	3 oz cooked	5	13	223
	1 lb raw	13	33	549
point half, all grades, braised	3 oz cooked	4	7	181
	1 lb raw	11	19	461

CHUCK, ARM POT ROAST

Lean & Fat

	Portion	Calcium (mg)	Total Fat (g)	Total Calor
all grades, braised	3 oz cooked	9	22	297
	1 lb raw	28	71	962
choice, braised	3 oz cooked	9	23	301
	1 lb raw	28	73	982
good, braised	3 oz cooked	9	21	287
	1 lb raw	27	65	894
prime, braised	3 oz cooked	9	26	332
	1 lb raw	29	86	1,082

Lean Only

	Portion	Calcium (mg)	Total Fat (g)	Total Calor
all grades, braised	3 oz cooked	7	8	196
	1 lb raw	18	20	467
choice, braised	3 oz cooked	7	7	199
	1 lb raw	18	18	473
good, braised	3 oz cooked	7	8	189
	1 lb raw	17	18	439
prime, braised	3 oz cooked	7	11	222
	1 lb raw	17	26	499

	Portion	Calcium (mg)	Total Fat (g)	Total Calor
CHUCK, BLADE ROAST				
Lean & Fat				
all grades, braised	3 oz cooked	11	26	325
	1 lb raw	32	76	961
choice, braised	3 oz cooked	11	26	330
	1 lb raw	33	78	982
good, braised	3 oz cooked	11	24	311
	1 lb raw	31	68	882
prime, braised	3 oz cooked	11	29	354
	1 lb raw	32	84	1,029
Lean Only				
all grades, braised	3 oz cooked	11	13	230
	1 lb raw	23	28	492
choice, braised	3 oz cooked	11	13	234
	1 lb raw	23	29	503
good, braised	3 oz cooked	11	12	218
	1 lb raw	22	24	456
prime, braised	3 oz cooked	11	17	270
	1 lb raw	22	37	569
FLANK				
Lean & Fat				
choice				
braised	3 oz cooked	6	13	218
	1 lb raw	18	41	689
broiled	3 oz cooked	5	14	216
	1 lb raw	21	55	863
Lean Only				
choice				
braised	3 oz cooked	6	12	208
	1 lb raw	17	36	635
broiled	3 oz cooked	5	13	207
	1 lb raw	20	50	808
GROUND BEEF				
Extra Lean				
baked				
medium	3 oz cooked	6	14	213
	1 lb raw	23	56	863
well done	3 oz cooked	7	14	232
	1 lb raw	23	43	733
broiled				
medium	3 oz cooked	6	14	217
	1 lb raw	25	55	859
well done	3 oz cooked	7	13	225
	1 lb raw	24	44	744

	Portion	Calcium (mg)	Total Fat (g)	Total Calor
pan-fried				
medium	3 oz cooked	6	14	216
	1 lb raw	24	56	866
well done	3 oz cooked	7	14	224
	1 lb raw	24	47	777
Lean				
baked				
medium	3 oz cooked	8	16	227
	1 lb raw	32	62	899
well done	3 oz cooked	10	16	248
	1 lb raw	32	48	768
broiled				
medium	3 oz cooked	9	16	231
	1 lb raw	34	59	876
well done	3 oz cooked	10	15	238
	1 lb raw	34	50	785
pan-fried				
medium	3 oz cooked	8	16	234
	1 lb raw	32	62	901
well done	3 oz cooked	9	15	235
	1 lb raw	31	51	791
Regular				
baked				
medium	3 oz cooked	8	18	244
	1 lb raw	31	67	913
well done	3 oz cooked	10	18	269
	1 lb raw	31	55	804
broiled				
medium	3 oz cooked	9	18	246
	1 lb raw	33	63	880
well done	3 oz cooked	10	17	248
	1 lb raw	33	53	793
pan-fried				
medium	3 oz cooked	10	19	260
	1 lb raw	34	69	941
well done	3 oz cooked	11	16	243
	1 lb raw	35	52	792
GROUND, FROZEN PATTIES				
broiled, medium	3 oz cooked	9	17	240
	1 lb raw	33	62	882
RIB, WHOLE (RIBS 6–12)				
Lean & Fat				
all grades				
broiled	3 oz cooked	10	25	308
	1 lb raw	33	86	1,039

	Portion	Calcium (mg)	Total Fat (g)	Total Calor
roasted	3 oz cooked	10	27	324
	1 lb raw	30	87	1,042
choice				
broiled	3 oz cooked	10	26	313
	1 lb raw	33	88	1,060
roasted	3 oz cooked	10	28	328
	1 lb raw	31	89	1,062
good				
broiled	3 oz cooked	9	23	289
	1 lb raw	31	78	969
roasted	3 oz cooked	10	25	306
	1 lb raw	30	80	978
prime				
broiled	3 oz cooked	10	30	347
	1 lb raw	34	104	1,199
roasted	3 oz cooked	10	31	361
	1 lb raw	31	103	1,189
Lean Only				
all grades				
broiled	3 oz cooked	9	11	194
	1 lb raw	21	26	461
roasted	3 oz cooked	9	12	204
	1 lb raw	18	26	449
choice				
broiled	3 oz cooked	9	12	198
	1 lb raw	21	27	469
roasted	3 oz cooked	9	12	209
	1 lb raw	18	27	456
good				
broiled	3 oz cooked	9	10	181
	1 lb raw	21	23	440
roasted	3 oz cooked	9	10	191
	1 lb raw	19	23	430
prime				
broiled	3 oz cooked	9	16	238
	1 lb raw	21	38	562
roasted	3 oz cooked	9	17	248
	1 lb raw	18	36	536

RIB, EYE, SMALL END (RIBS 10–12)

Lean & Fat

	Portion	Calcium (mg)	Total Fat (g)	Total Calor
choice, broiled	3 oz cooked	11	18	250
	1 lb raw	43	68	966

Lean Only

	Portion	Calcium (mg)	Total Fat (g)	Total Calor
choice, broiled	3 oz cooked	11	10	191
	1 lb raw	36	32	623

	Portion	Calcium (mg)	Total Fat (g)	Total Calor
RIB, LARGE END (RIBS 6–9)				
Lean & Fat				
all grades				
broiled	3 oz cooked	9	27	321
	1 lb raw	29	93	1,083
roasted	3 oz cooked	8	26	313
	1 lb raw	27	84	1,030
choice				
broiled	3 oz cooked	9	28	327
	1 lb raw	30	95	1,107
roasted	3 oz cooked	8	26	316
	1 lb raw	27	85	1,040
good				
broiled	3 oz cooked	9	25	301
	1 lb raw	29	84	1,009
roasted	3 oz cooked	8	24	304
	1 lb raw	27	81	1,000
prime				
broiled	3 oz cooked	9	32	361
	1 lb raw	31	112	1,267
roasted	3 oz cooked	8	29	346
	1 lb raw	27	97	1,136
Lean Only				
all grades				
broiled	3 oz cooked	7	12	198
	1 lb raw	16	28	453
roasted	3 oz cooked	7	12	207
	1 lb raw	16	28	487
choice				
broiled	3 oz cooked	7	13	203
	1 lb raw	16	29	464
roasted	3 oz cooked	7	12	210
	1 lb raw	16	29	495
good				
broiled	3 oz cooked	7	10	183
	1 lb raw	17	24	428
roasted	3 oz cooked	7	11	197
	1 lb raw	16	26	468
prime				
broiled	3 oz cooked	7	18	250
	1 lb raw	17	41	575
roasted	3 oz cooked	7	16	241
	1 lb raw	15	35	543

	Portion	Calcium (mg)	Total Fat (g)	Total Calor
RIB, SMALL END (RIBS 10–12)				
Lean & Fat				
all grades				
broiled	3 oz cooked	11	21	277
	1 lb raw	39	72	950
roasted	3 oz cooked	11	25	305
	1 lb raw	36	80	981
choice				
broiled	3 oz cooked	11	22	282
	1 lb raw	39	74	965
roasted	3 oz cooked	11	26	312
	1 lb raw	36	82	1,002
good				
broiled	3 oz cooked	11	19	263
	1 lb raw	38	66	889
roasted	3 oz cooked	11	22	283
	1 lb raw	36	71	900
prime				
broiled	3 oz cooked	11	25	309
	1 lb raw	38	83	1,041
roasted	3 oz cooked	11	31	357
	1 lb raw	36	99	1,142
Lean Only				
all grades				
broiled	3 oz cooked	11	10	188
	1 lb raw	29	25	492
roasted	3 oz cooked	11	11	201
	1 lb raw	26	27	465
choice				
broiled	3 oz cooked	11	10	191
	1 lb raw	29	26	499
roasted	3 oz cooked	11	12	206
	1 lb raw	26	28	476
good				
broiled	3 oz cooked	11	8	178
	1 lb raw	29	22	473
roasted	3 oz cooked	11	10	183
	1 lb raw	26	23	433
prime				
broiled	3 oz cooked	11	13	221
	1 lb raw	28	33	559
roasted	3 oz cooked	11	18	259
	1 lb raw	25	40	572
RIB, SHORT				
Lean & Fat				
choice, braised	3 oz cooked	10	36	400
	1 lb raw	28	95	1,064

	Portion	Calcium (mg)	Total Fat (g)	Total Calor
Lean Only				
choice, braised	3 oz cooked	9	15	251
	1 lb raw	13	22	363
ROUND, FULL CUT				
Lean & Fat				
choice, broiled	3 oz cooked	6	16	233
	1 lb raw	21	55	832
good, broiled	3 oz cooked	6	14	222
	1 lb raw	20	51	790
Lean Only				
choice, broiled	3 oz cooked	5	7	165
	1 lb raw	14	20	493
good, broiled	3 oz cooked	5	6	157
	1 lb raw	14	18	470
ROUND, BOTTOM				
Lean & Fat				
all grades, braised	3 oz cooked	5	13	222
	1 lb raw	16	41	725
choice, braised	3 oz cooked	5	13	224
	1 lb raw	16	42	734
good, braised	3 oz cooked	5	12	215
	1 lb raw	16	38	700
prime, braised	3 oz cooked	5	16	253
	1 lb raw	17	59	853
Lean Only				
all grades, braised	3 oz cooked	4	8	189
	1 lb raw	12	25	564
choice, braised	3 oz cooked	4	8	191
	1 lb raw	12	25	571
good, braised	3 oz cooked	4	7	182
	1 lb raw	12	22	543
prime, braised	3 oz cooked	4	11	212
	1 lb raw	12	32	622
ROUND, EYE OF				
Lean & Fat				
all grades, roasted	3 oz cooked	5	12	206
	1 lb raw	20	51	869
choice, roasted	3 oz cooked	5	12	207
	1 lb raw	20	51	871
good, roasted	3 oz cooked	5	12	201
	1 lb raw	20	49	851
prime, roasted	3 oz cooked	5	13	213
	1 lb raw	20	53	888

	Portion	Calcium (mg)	Total Fat (g)	Total Calor
Lean Only				
all grades, roasted	3 oz cooked	4	6	155
	1 lb raw	14	21	575
choice, roasted	3 oz cooked	4	6	156
	1 lb raw	14	21	578
good, roasted	3 oz cooked	4	5	151
	1 lb raw	14	19	562
prime, roasted	3 oz cooked	4	7	168
	1 lb raw	14	26	628
ROUND, TIP				
Lean & Fat				
all grades, roasted	3 oz cooked	6	13	213
	1 lb raw	21	50	823
choice, roasted	3 oz cooked	6	13	216
	1 lb raw	21	52	837
good, roasted	3 oz cooked	5	12	205
	1 lb raw	21	46	780
prime, roasted	3 oz cooked	6	16	242
	1 lb raw	22	63	932
Lean Only				
all grades, roasted	3 oz cooked	5	6	162
	1 lb raw	16	22	546
choice, roasted	3 oz cooked	5	7	164
	1 lb raw	16	22	552
good, roasted	3 oz cooked	5	6	156
	1 lb raw	16	19	524
prime, roasted	3 oz cooked	5	9	181
	1 lb raw	15	28	593
ROUND, TOP				
Lean & Fat				
all grades, broiled	3 oz cooked	5	7	179
	1 lb raw	21	29	701
choice				
broiled	3 oz cooked	5	8	181
	1 lb raw	21	30	709
pan-fried	3 oz cooked	5	15	246
	1 lb raw	18	48	819
good, broiled	3 oz cooked	5	7	176
	1 lb raw	21	28	686
prime, broiled	3 oz cooked	5	10	201
	1 lb raw	21	39	783
Lean Only				
all grades, broiled	3 oz cooked	5	5	162
	1 lb raw	19	20	610

	Portion	Calcium (mg)	Total Fat (g)	Total Calor
choice				
broiled	3 oz cooked	5	5	165
	1 lb raw	19	21	617
pan-fried	3 oz cooked	4	7	193
	1, lb raw	12	21	556
good, broiled	3 oz cooked	5	5	156
	1 lb raw	19	17	583
prime, broiled	3 oz cooked	5	8	183
	1 lb raw	19	28	678

SHANK CROSSCUTS
Lean & Fat

	Portion	Calcium (mg)	Total Fat (g)	Total Calor
choice, simmered	3 oz cooked	26	10	208
	1 lb raw	63	25	508

Lean Only

	Portion	Calcium (mg)	Total Fat (g)	Total Calor
choice, simmered	3 oz cooked	27	5	171
	1 lb raw	60	12	380

SHORT LOIN, PORTERHOUSE STEAK
Lean & Fat

	Portion	Calcium (mg)	Total Fat (g)	Total Calor
choice, broiled	3 oz cooked	7	18	254
	1 lb raw	23	57	803

Lean Only

	Portion	Calcium (mg)	Total Fat (g)	Total Calor
choice, broiled	3 oz cooked	6	9	185
	1 lb raw	16	24	483

SHORT LOIN, T-BONE STEAK
Lean & Fat

	Portion	Calcium (mg)	Total Fat (g)	Total Calor
choice, broiled	3 oz cooked	8	21	276
	1 lb raw	24	67	888

Lean Only

	Portion	Calcium (mg)	Total Fat (g)	Total Calor
choice, broiled	3 oz cooked	6	9	182
	1 lb raw	15	22	447

SHORT LOIN, TENDERLOIN
Lean & Fat

	Portion	Calcium (mg)	Total Fat (g)	Total Calor
all grades				
broiled	3 oz cooked	7	15	226
	1 raw steak, edible portion = 4 oz	9	20	306
roasted	3 oz cooked	7	19	258
	1 raw steak, edible portion = 4.2 oz	10	26	364

	Portion	Calcium (mg)	Total Fat (g)	Total Calor
choice				
broiled	3 oz cooked	6	15	230
	1 raw steak, edible portion = 4.1 oz	9	21	314
roasted	3 oz cooked	7	19	262
	1 raw steak, edible portion = 4.2 oz	10	27	370
good				
broiled	3 oz cooked	6	13	216
	1 raw steak, edible portion = 4 oz	9	18	286
roasted	3 oz cooked	7	17	245
	1 raw steak, edible portion = 4.2 oz	10	24	343
prime				
broiled	3 oz cooked	7	20	270
	1 raw steak, edible portion = 4 oz	9	27	362
roasted	3 oz cooked	7	24	305
	1 raw steak, edible portion = 4.1 oz	10	33	416
Lean Only				
all grades				
broiled	3 oz cooked	6	8	174
	1 raw steak, edible portion = 3½ oz	7	9	204
roasted	3 oz cooked	6	10	186
	1 raw steak, edible portion = 3½ oz	7	11	215
choice				
broiled	3 oz cooked	6	8	176
	1 raw steak, edible portion = 3.6 oz	7	10	209

	Portion	Calcium (mg)	Total Fat (g)	Total Calor
choice *(cont.)*				
roasted	3 oz cooked	6	10	189
	1 raw steak, edible portion = 3.4 oz	7	11	216
good				
broiled	3 oz cooked	6	7	167
	1 raw steak, edible portion = 3½ oz	7	8	196
roasted	3 oz cooked	6	9	177
	1 raw steak, edible portion = 3½ oz	7	10	206
prime				
broiled	3 oz cooked	6	11	197
	1 raw steak, edible portion = 3.2 oz	6	11	214
roasted	3 oz cooked	6	13	217
	1 raw steak, edible portion = 3.1 oz	6	13	225
SHORT LOIN, TOP				
Lean & Fat				
all grades, broiled	3 oz cooked	7	16	238
	1 raw steak, edible portion = 8.2 oz	21	44	651
choice, broiled	3 oz cooked	8	17	243
	1 raw steak, edible portion = 8.3 oz	21	46	672
good, broiled	3 oz cooked	7	14	223
	1 raw steak, edible portion = 8.1 oz	20	39	603

	Portion	Calcium (mg)	Total Fat (g)	Total Calor
prime, broiled	3 oz cooked	8	22	288
	1 raw steak, edible portion = 8.1 oz	21	59	774
Lean Only				
all grades, broiled	3 oz cooked	7	8	172
	1 raw steak, edible portion = 6.9 oz	15	17	395
choice, broiled	3 oz cooked	7	8	176
	1 raw steak, edible portion = 6.9 oz	15	18	406
good, broiled	3 oz cooked	7	6	162
	1 raw steak, edible portion = 6.9 oz	15	15	373
prime, broiled	3 oz cooked	7	12	208
	1 raw steak, edible portion = 6.3 oz	14	24	438
WEDGE-BONE SIRLOIN				
Lean & Fat				
all grades, broiled	3 oz cooked	9	15	238
	1 lb raw	31	51	791
choice				
broiled	3 oz cooked	9	16	240
	1 lb raw	31	52	804
pan-fried	3 oz cooked	10	21	288
	1 lb raw	31	66	913
good, broiled	3 oz cooked	9	15	232
	1 lb raw	31	49	777
prime, broiled	3 oz cooked	9	19	271
	1 lb raw	31	63	878
Lean Only				
all grades, broiled	3 oz cooked	9	7	177
	1 lb raw	25	21	500
choice				
broiled	3 oz cooked	9	8	180
	1 lb raw	25	22	509
pan-fried	3 oz cooked	9	9	202
	1 lb raw	22	23	492

	Portion	Calcium (mg)	Total Fat (g)	Total Calor
good, broiled	3 oz cooked	9	7	170
	1 lb raw	25	19	482
prime, broiled	3 oz cooked	9	10	201
	1 lb raw	23	26	527

VARIETY MEATS

brains				
pan-fried	3 oz cooked	8	13	167
	1 lb raw	32	56	690
simmered	3 oz cooked	8	11	136
	1 lb raw	36	49	627
heart, simmered	3 oz cooked	5	5	148
	1 lb raw	16	14	450
kidneys, simmered	3 oz cooked	15	3	122
	1 lb raw	34	7	283
liver				
braised	3 oz cooked	6	4	137
	1 lb raw	23	16	542
pan-fried	3 oz cooked	9	7	184
	1 lb raw	31	24	639
lungs, braised	3 oz cooked	9	3	102
	1 lb raw	33	11	365
suet, raw	1 oz	?	27	242
tongue, simmered	3 oz cooked	6	18	241
	1 lb raw	19	54	732
tripe, raw	1 oz	?	1	28
	4 oz	?	4	111

Beef, Cured

breakfast strips, cooked	3 (15 per 12 oz pkg)	?	12	153
	6 oz	?	58	764
corned beef brisket, braised	3 oz cooked	7	16	213
	1 lb raw	25	61	802

- **BRAND NAME**

Oscar Mayer

breakfast strips, cooked	1 (15 per 12 oz pkg)	1	4	46

❑ BEVERAGES
See also FAST FOODS; MILK, MILK SUBSTITUTES, & MILK PRODUCTS

	Portion	Calcium (mg)	Total Fat (g)	Total Calor

Beverages, Alcoholic

BEER & ALE

	Portion	Calcium (mg)	Total Fat (g)	Total Calor
ale, mild	8 fl oz	30	0	98
beer				
regular (alcohol 4½% by volume)	12 fl oz	18	0	146
light (alcohol content of light beer varies)	12 fl oz	18	0	100

COCKTAILS & MIXED DRINKS

	Portion	Calcium (mg)	Total Fat (g)	Total Calor
Bloody Mary	5 fl oz	10	tr	116
bourbon & soda	4 fl oz	4	0	105
daiquiri, canned	6.8 fl oz	1	?	?
daiquiri cocktail	2 fl oz	2	0	111
eggnog See Flavored Milk Beverages, *below*				
gin & tonic	7½ fl oz	4	0	171
Gin Rickey	4 fl oz	2	?	150
manhattan	2 fl oz	1	0	128
martini	2½ fl oz	1	0	156
piña colada, canned	6.8 fl oz	1	17	525
piña colada cocktail	4½ fl oz	11	3	262
planter's punch	3½ fl oz	4	?	175
screwdriver	7 fl oz	16	tr	174
tequila sunrise, canned	6.8 fl oz	1	?	?
tequila sunrise cocktail	5½ fl oz	10	tr	189
Tom Collins	7½ fl oz	10	0	121
whiskey sour, canned	6.8 fl oz	1	?	?
whiskey sour cocktail	3 fl oz	5	tr	123
whiskey sour mix				
powder	1 pkt	45	0	64
prepared w/water & whiskey	1 pkt + 1½ fl oz water + 1½ fl oz whiskey	47	0	169
bottled (no alcohol)	2 fl oz	1	0	55
prepared w/whiskey	2 fl oz mix + 1½ fl oz whiskey	1	0	158

CORDIALS & LIQUEURS

	Portion	Calcium (mg)	Total Fat (g)	Total Calor
54 proof (22.1% alcohol by weight)	1 fl oz	0	0	97
coffee liqueur (53 proof)	1½ fl oz	1	tr	174
coffee w/cream liqueur (34 proof)	1½ fl oz	7	7	154
crème de menthe liqueur (72 proof)	1½ fl oz	0	tr	186

	Portion	Calcium (mg)	Total Fat (g)	Total Calor
DISTILLED SPIRITS				
all (gin, rum, vodka, whiskey)				
100 proof	1 fl oz	0	0	82
	1½ fl oz	0	0	124
94 proof	1 fl oz	0	0	76
	1½ fl oz	0	0	116
gin, 90 proof	1½ fl oz	0	0	110
rum, 80 proof	1½ fl oz	0	0	97
vodka, 80 proof	1½ fl oz	0	0	97
whiskey, 86 proof	1½ fl oz	0	0	105
WINES				
champagne	4 fl oz	?	?	84
dessert wine, sweet, 18.8% alcohol by volume	1 fl oz	2	0	46
muscatel or port	3½ fl oz	8	?	158
sauterne	3½ fl oz	?	?	84
sherry	2 fl oz	5	?	84
table wine, 11½% alcohol by volume				
red	1 fl oz	2	0	21
	3½ fl oz	8	0	74
rosé	1 fl oz	2	0	21
	3½ fl oz	9	0	73
white	1 fl oz	3	0	20
	3½ fl oz	9	0	70
vermouth, dry, French	3½ fl oz	8	?	105

Beverages, Carbonated

	Portion	Calcium (mg)	Total Fat (g)	Total Calor
bitter lemon	12 fl oz	?	0	192
club soda	12 fl oz	17	0	0
cola	12 fl oz	9	tr	151
low-cal, aspartame-sweetened	12 fl oz	12	0	2
low-cal, sodium-saccharin-sweetened	12 fl oz	14	0	2
cream soda	12 fl oz	19	0	191
diet soda, all flavors	12 fl oz	14	0	0
ginger ale	12 fl oz	12	0	124
grape soda	12 fl oz	12	0	161
lemon-lime soda	12 fl oz	9	0	149
orange soda	12 fl oz	19	0	177
peach soda	12 fl oz	0	0	184
quinine water	4 fl oz	12	0	37
root beer	12 fl oz	19	0	152
diet	12 fl oz	?	0	1

	Portion	Calcium (mg)	Total Fat (g)	Total Calor
strawberry soda	12 fl oz	0	0	174
tonic water	12 fl oz	5	0	125

Coffee & Coffee Substitutes

coffee, brewed	6 fl oz	3	0	4
coffee, instant, regular or de-caffeinated, powder, pre-pared w/water	6 fl oz water + 1 rounded t powder	6	0	4
coffee substitute, cereal grain beverage, powder				
prepared w/water	6 fl oz water + 1 t pow-der	5	tr	9
prepared w/whole milk	6 fl oz milk + 1 t pow-der	219	6	121

Flavored Milk Beverages

carob-flavored mix				
powder	3 t	?	0	45
powder, prepared w/whole milk	1 c milk + 3 t powder	291	8	195
chocolate dairy drink, re-duced-calorie, aspartame-sweetened, powder, pre-pared w/water	½ c water + 3 ice cubes + ¾ oz pkt	192	1	64
chocolate-flavored mix				
powder	2–3 heaping t	8	1	75
powder, prepared w/whole milk	1 c milk + 2–3 heaping t powder	300	9	226
chocolate milk				
whole	1 c	280	8	208
low-fat, 2%	1 c	284	5	179
low-fat, 1%	1 c	287	3	158
chocolate syrup				
w/added nutrients	1 T	?	tr	46
prepared w/whole milk	1 c milk + 1 T syrup	292	8	196
w/out added nutrients	1 fl oz	5	tr	82
prepared w/whole milk	1 c milk + 2 T syrup	297	9	232
cocoa, homemade, w/whole milk	6 fl oz 1 c	224 298	7 9	164 218

	Portion	Calcium (mg)	Total Fat (g)	Total Calor
cocoa mix				
reduced-calorie, aspartame-sweetened, powder, prepared w/water	6 fl oz water + .53 oz pkt	90	tr	48
w/added nutrients	6 fl oz water + 1 pkt	104	3	120
w/out added nutrients	6 fl oz water + 3–4 heaping t powder	96	1	103
eggnog, dairy	1 c	330	19	342
eggnog-flavored mix, powder, prepared w/whole milk	1 c milk + 2 heaping t powder	291	8	260
malt beverage	12 fl oz	25	0	32
malted milk–flavored mix, chocolate				
w/added nutrients				
powder	¾ oz or 4–5 heaping t	93	1	75
powder, prepared w/whole milk	1 c milk + 4–5 heaping t powder	384	9	225
w/out added nutrients				
powder	¾ oz or 3 heaping t	13	1	79
powder prepared w/whole milk	1 c milk + 3 heaping t powder	304	9	229
malted milk–flavored mix, natural				
w/added nutrients				
powder	¾ oz or 4–5 heaping t	79	1	80
powder, prepared w/whole milk	1 c milk + 4–5 heaping t powder	370	9	230
w/out added nutrients				
powder	¾ oz or 3 heaping t	63	2	87
powder, prepared w/whole milk	1 c milk + 3 heaping t powder	354	10	237
shake, thick				
chocolate	10.6 oz	396	8	356
vanilla	about 11 oz	457	9	350
strawberry-flavored mix, powder, prepared w/whole milk	1 c milk + 2–3 heaping t powder	292	8	234

	Portion	Calcium (mg)	Total Fat (g)	Total Calor
Fruit & Vegetable Juices				
acerola	1 c	24	1	51
apple				
canned or bottled	1 c	16	tr	116
from frozen concentrate	1 c	14	tr	111
apricot, canned	1 c	17	tr	141
carrot, canned	½ c	29	tr	49
cranberry, bottled	1 c	8	tr	147
grape				
canned	1 c	22	tr	155
from frozen concentrate, sweetened	1 c	9	tr	128
grapefruit				
fresh	1 c	22	tr	96
canned				
sweetened	1 c	20	tr	116
unsweetened	1 c	18	tr	93
from frozen concentrate	1 c	19	tr	102
lemon				
fresh	1 T	1	0	4
canned or bottled	1 T	2	tr	3
frozen, single strength	1 T	1	tr	3
lime				
fresh	1 T	1	tr	4
canned or bottled	1 T	2	tr	3
orange				
fresh	1 c	27	1	111
canned	1 c	21	tr	104
from frozen concentrate	1 c	22	tr	112
frozen concentrate, undiluted	6 fl oz	67	tr	339
orange-grapefruit, canned	1 c	21	tr	107
papaya, canned	1 c	24	tr	142
passion fruit				
purple	1 c	9	tr	126
yellow	1 c	9	tr	149
peach, canned	1 c	13	tr	134
pear, canned	1 c	11	tr	149
pineapple				
canned	1 c	42	tr	139
from frozen concentrate	1 c	28	tr	129
prune, canned	1 c	30	tr	181
tangerine				
fresh	1 c	44	tr	106
canned, sweetened	1 c	45	1	125
from frozen concentrate, sweetened	1 c	18	tr	110
tomato, canned	6 fl oz	16	tr	32
w/beef broth	5½ fl oz	19	tr	61
w/clam juice	5½ fl oz	21	tr	77
vegetable, canned	6 fl oz	20	tr	34

	Portion	Calcium (mg)	Total Fat (g)	Total Calor
Fruit Juice Drinks (10–50% Fruit Juice), Juice Ades, & Juice-flavored Drinks & Powders				
apple juice drink, canned	6 fl oz	13	tr	92
cherry juice drink, canned	6 fl oz	?	tr	93
citrus fruit drink, canned	6 fl oz	?	tr	93
citrus fruit juice drink, from frozen concentrate	1 c	21	0	114
cranberry-apple juice drink				
bottled	6 fl oz	13	0	123
canned	6 fl oz	10	1	135
cranberry-apricot juice drink, bottled	6 fl oz	17	0	118
cranberry-grape juice drink, bottled	6 fl oz	15	tr	103
cranberry juice cocktail				
bottled	6 fl oz	7	tr	108
from frozen concentrate	6 fl oz	9	0	102
low-cal, calcium-saccharin- & corn-sweetened, bottled	6 fl oz	16	0	33
Florida punch juice drink, canned	6 fl oz	?	tr	95
fruit juice drink, from mix, average for 9 flavors	6 fl oz	25	tr	70
fruit punch drink				
canned	6 fl oz	14	0	87
from frozen concentrate	1 c	9	0	113
fruit punch–flavored drink, powder, prepared w/water	1 c water + 2 rounded T powder	41	0	97
fruit punch juice drink				
canned	6 fl oz	6	tr	99
from frozen concentrate	1 c	18	1	123
gelatin drink, orange-flavored, powder	0.6 oz pkt	?	tr	67
grape drink, canned	6 fl oz	?	0	84
grape juice drink, canned	6 fl oz	6	0	94
lemonade				
from frozen concentrate	1 c	8	tr	100
powder, prepared w/water	1 c water + 2 T powder	71	0	102
powder, low-cal, aspartame-sweetened	0.42 oz pkt	369	0	40
	0.67 oz pkt	589	tr	63
lemonade-flavored drink, powder, prepared w/water	1 c water + 2 T powder	29	tr	113
lemon-lime, from mix	8 fl oz	tr	tr	91
limeade, from frozen concentrate	1 c	7	tr	102

	Portion	Calcium (mg)	Total Fat (g)	Total Calor
orange & apricot juice drink, canned	1 c	13	tr	128
orange drink, canned	6 fl oz	12	0	94
orange drink, breakfast type, from frozen concentrate (orange juice & orange pulp)	6 fl oz	221	0	84
orange-flavored drink, breakfast type				
from frozen concentrate w/ orange pulp	6 fl oz	61	tr	91
from powder	3 rounded t powder + 6 fl oz water	46	0	86
orange juice drink, canned	6 fl oz	?	tr	92
orange-pineapple juice drink, canned	6 fl oz	?	tr	94
peach juice drink, canned	6 fl oz	2	tr	90
pineapple & grapefruit juice drink, canned	1 c	18	tr	117
pineapple & orange juice drink, canned	1 c	13	0	125
pineapple-orange juice drink, canned	6 fl oz	9	0	99
strawberry juice drink, canned	6 fl oz	?	tr	89
tangerine juice drink, canned	6 fl oz	2	tr	90
wild berry juice drink, canned	6 fl oz	?	tr	88

Tea

	Portion	Calcium (mg)	Total Fat (g)	Total Calor
brewed	6 fl oz	0	0	2
herb, brewed	6 fl oz	4	0	1
iced, canned, sweetened	12 fl oz	?	0	146
instant, powder				
low-cal, sodium-saccharin-sweetened, lemon-flavored	2 t	0	0	5
sugar-sweetened, lemon-flavored	3 rounded t	6	tr	87
sweetened	3 t in 8 fl oz water	1	tr	86
unsweetened	1 t	5	0	2
unsweetened, lemon-flavored	1 rounded t	5	0	4

	Portion	Calcium (mg)	Total Fat (g)	Total Calor
Water				
municipal (mineral content will vary depending on water source)	1 c	5	0	0

• BRAND NAME

NOTE: Brand-name carbonated soft drinks for which calcium values are available contain 0 to trace amounts of calcium except for Sprite, below.

	Portion	Calcium (mg)	Total Fat (g)	Total Calor
Apple & Eve Juices				
apple	6 fl oz	9	tr	75
apple cranberry	6 fl oz	13	tr	75
apple grape	6 fl oz	13	tr	83
cranberry-grape	6 fl oz	17	tr	94
raspberry-cranberry	6 fl oz	22	tr	86
vegetable	6 fl oz	12	tr	34
Awake				
from frozen concentrate	6 fl oz	59	tr	91
Bright & Early				
imitation orange beverage, from carton or frozen concentrate	6 fl oz	?	1	90
Campbell Juices				
apple	6 oz	20	0	100
appleberry	6 oz	20	0	100
cherry	6 oz	<20	0	100
grape	6 oz	<20	0	100
orange	6 oz	<20	0	90
strawberry	6 oz	40	0	100
tomato	6 oz	<20	0	35
Country Time Drink Mix				
all	8 fl oz	<20	?	varies
Crystal Light Drink Mix				
all	8 fl oz	<20	?	4
Dole Juices				
pineapple	6 oz	28	tr	103
pineapple–pink grapefruit	6 oz	9	tr	101
New pineapple	6 oz	?	tr	100
New pineapple-grapefruit	6 oz	?	tr	90
New pineapple-orange	6 oz	?	tr	100

	Portion	Calcium (mg)	Total Fat (g)	Total Calor
Five Alive Fruit Drinks				
CARTONS				
berry citrus	6 fl oz	3	tr	88
citrus	6 fl oz	9	tr	87
tropical citrus	6 fl oz	8	tr	88
FROZEN CONCENTRATE				
berry citrus	6 fl oz	3	tr	88
citrus	6 fl oz	8	tr	87
fruit punch	6 fl oz	8	tr	87
tropical citrus	6 fl oz	8	tr	85
Gatorade				
lemon-lime or orange flavor, w/water	8 fl oz	<20	0	60
Hawaiian Punch				
Hawaiian Punch, canned	8 fl oz	20	tr	120
Hershey				
chocolate-flavored syrup	2 T	<20	1	80
chocolate milk, 2% low-fat	1 c	300	5	190
cocoa	⅓ c	40	4	120
instant cocoa	3 T	<20	1	80
Hi-C Fruit Drinks				
Double Fruit Cooler	6 fl oz	1	tr	86
fruit punch	6 fl oz	12	tr	92
100 Apple	6 fl oz	11	tr	89
100 Grape	6 fl oz	13	tr	94
100 Orange	6 fl oz	21	tr	94
International Coffees				
all regular	6 oz	<20	2–3	50–60
all sugar-free	6 oz	<20	2–3	25–35
Kool-Aid				
KOOLERS				
all	8.45 fl oz	<20	0	130
SOFT DRINK MIX				
Sugar-free				
grape	8 fl oz	60	0	4
Mountain Berry punch	8 fl oz	20	0	4
Rainbow punch	8 fl oz	20	0	4
Tropical punch	8 fl oz	20	0	4
Sugar-sweetened				
grape	8 fl oz	<20	0	80
Rainbow punch	8 fl oz	20	0	80
Tropical punch	8 fl oz	<20	0	80

	Portion	Calcium (mg)	Total Fat (g)	Total Calor
Unsweetened, Prepared w/Sugar				
Rainbow punch, Sunshine punch, Tropical punch	8 fl oz	20	0	100
Land O'Lakes				
chocolate milk				
homogenized	8 fl oz	300	8	210
1% low-fat	8 fl oz	300	3	160
skim	8 fl oz	300	<1	140
eggnog	8 fl oz	300	15	300
fruit-flavored drinks	8 fl oz	<20	0	120
Light 'n Juicy Juice Drinks				
grape, carton	6 fl oz	2	0	12
lemonade, carton	6 fl oz	2	tr	5
orange, carton	6 fl oz	2	tr	14
punch, carton	6 fl oz	2	0	12
Minute Maid				
FRUIT ADES				
grapeade, carton or from frozen concentrate	6 fl oz	3	0	94
lemonade or pink lemonade				
carton	6 fl oz	2	tr	81
from frozen concentrate	6 fl oz	2	tr	77
lemon/limeade, from frozen concentrate	6 fl oz	2	tr	77
orangeade, from frozen concentrate	6 fl oz	3	tr	85
FRUIT JUICES				
apple, carton or from frozen concentrate	6 fl oz	1	tr	90
fruit punch, carton or from frozen concentrate	6 fl oz	1	0	91
grape, sweetened, from frozen concentrate	6 fl oz	14	0	98
grapefruit				
carton	6 fl oz	17	tr	65
from frozen concentrate	6 fl oz	10	tr	71
grapefruit, pink, from frozen concentrate	6 fl oz	18	tr	71
lemon juice, from frozen concentrate	6 fl oz	13	tr	22
orange				
regular, carton or from frozen concentrate	6 fl oz	17	tr	82
calcium-fortified, carton or from frozen concentrate	6 fl oz	320	tr	84
Country Style, carton or from frozen concentrate	6 fl oz	17	tr	82

	Portion	Calcium (mg)	Total Fat (g)	Total Calor
reduced-acid, from frozen concentrate	6 fl oz	17	tr	82
pineapple, from frozen concentrate	6 fl oz	20	tr	93
pineapple orange, from frozen concentrate	6 fl oz	19	tr	91
tangerine, sweetened, from frozen concentrate	6 fl oz	27	tr	82
Mott's				
JUICES				
apple	6 oz	11	0	88
apple, natural	6 oz	31	0	76
apple cranberry	6 oz	24	0	83
apple grape	6 oz	28	0	86
apple raspberry	6 oz	28	0	83
grapefruit	10 oz	25	0	124
prune				
regular	6 oz	19	0	130
Country Style	6 oz	22	0	130
JUICE DRINKS				
apple cranberry drink	10 oz	6	0	176
apple raspberry drink	10 oz	10	0	158
Beefamato	6 oz	17	0	80
Clamato	6 oz	23	0	96
fruit punch	10 oz	?	0	170
grape apple drink	10 oz	1	0	167
orange fruit juice blend	10 oz	26	0	144
Orange Plus				
from frozen concentrate	6 fl oz	41	tr	97
Ortega				
Snap-E-Tom tomato cocktail	6 fl oz	20	0	40
Ovaltine Drink Mixes				
chocolate & malt	¾ oz dry mix	48	tr	80
	¾ oz dry mix + 8 oz 2% milk	630	5	200
cocoa				
Hot 'n Rich	1 oz or 5 t	100	3	120
50-calorie	0.45 oz or about 2½ t	100	2	50
sugar-free	0.41 oz or about 2½ t	100	1	40
PDQ Drink Mixes				
chocolate	3–4 t + 8 oz whole milk	290	5	180
eggnog	2–3 t + 8 oz whole milk	290	5	230

	Portion	Calcium (mg)	Total Fat (g)	Total Calor
strawberry	3–4 t + 8 oz whole milk	290	5	180
Perrier				
water, bottled	8 fl oz	33	0	0
Poland Spring				
water, bottled	1 c	3	0	0
Postum				
instant hot beverage, regular or coffee-flavored	6 fl oz	<20	0	12
Sprite				
soda	12 fl oz	11	?	144
Sunrise				
flavored instant coffee	0.07 oz + 6 fl oz water	?	tr	6
Tang				
grape	3 rounded t in 6 fl oz water	40	0	89
grapefruit	3 rounded t in 6 fl oz water	40	0	87
orange	3 rounded t in 6 fl oz water	40	tr	89
V8				
vegetable juice				
regular	6 oz	20	0	35
no salt added	6 oz	20	0	40
Spicy Hot V8	6 oz	20	0	35

❑ BISCUITS *See* BREADS, ROLLS, BISCUITS, & MUFFINS

❑ BREADCRUMBS, CROUTONS, STUFFINGS, & SEASONED COATINGS

	Portion	Calcium (mg)	Total Fat (g)	Total Calor
breadcrumbs				
enriched, dry, grated	1 c	122	5	390
white bread, enriched, soft	1 c	57	2	120
bread cubes, white, enriched	1 c	38	1	80
cornflake crumbs	1 oz	1	0	110
croutons, herb-seasoned	0.7 oz	20	0	70
stuffing, from mix				
bread	½ c	38	12	198

	Portion	Calcium (mg)	Total Fat (g)	Total Calor
corn bread	½ c	45	23	117
enriched bread				
dry type	1 c	92	31	500
moist type	1 c	81	26	420

▪ BRAND NAME

Kellogg's
cornflake crumbs	1 oz	1	0	110
Croutettes	0.7 oz dry	20	0	70

Nabisco
cracker meal	2 T	<20	0	50

Pepperidge Farm
CROUTONS
cheese & garlic	½ oz	20	3	70
onion & garlic	½ oz	<20	3	70
seasoned	½ oz	20	3	70

STUFFINGS
corn bread	1 oz	20	1	110
cube	1 oz	20	1	110
herb-seasoned	1 oz	40	1	110

Pillsbury Stuffing Originals
all	½ c	≤20	8	150–170

Rice-A-Roni Stuffing Mixes
bread/chicken flavor w/rice, prepared	½ c	<20	16	240
bread/herb & butter & wild rice, prepared	½ c	20	16	240
bread w/wild rice, prepared	½ c	20	16	240
corn bread w/rice, prepared	½ c	<20	16	240

Shake 'n Bake Seasoned Coatings
Extra Crispy
for chicken	¼ pouch	20	2	110
for pork	¼ pouch	<20	3	120
Homestyle for chicken	¼ pouch	<20	2	80

Stove Top
FLEXIBLE SERVING STUFFING MIX
chicken flavor, w/salted butter	½ c	20	9	170
corn bread flavor, w/salted butter	½ c	20	8	170
Homestyle herb, w/salted butter	½ c	40	9	170

	Portion	Calcium (mg)	Total Fat (g)	Total Calor
STUFFING MIX				
Americana New England, w/ salted butter	½ c	40	9	180
Americana San Francisco, w/ salted butter	½ c	20	9	170
beef, w/salted butter	½ c	20	9	180
chicken flavor, w/salted butter	½ c	20	9	180
corn bread, w/salted butter	½ c	20	9	170
long grain & wild rice, w/ salted butter	½ c	20	9	180
savory herbs, w/salted butter	½ c	40	9	180
turkey, w/salted butter	½ c	20	9	170
wild rice, w/salted butter	½ c	20	9	180

❑ BREADS, ROLLS, BISCUITS, & MUFFINS

Biscuits

	Portion	Calcium (mg)	Total Fat (g)	Total Calor
baking powder, prepared w/ vegetable shortening				
from mix	1 (2″ diam)	58	3	95
from refrigerator dough	1 (2″ diam)	4	2	65
homemade	1 (2″ diam)	47	5	100
buttermilk, from refrigerator dough	2	?	6	130
flaky, from refrigerator dough	2	?	9	180

Bread & Bread Sticks

	Portion	Calcium (mg)	Total Fat (g)	Total Calor
Boston brown bread, canned	1.6 oz slice	41	1	95
bread sticks				
regular	1	?	tr	23
Vienna	1	3	tr	18
coffee cake *See* DESSERTS: CAKES, PASTRIES, & PIES				
corn bread				
from mix	2 oz	?	4	160
homemade				
w/enriched cornmeal	2.9 oz	90	7	198
w/whole-ground cornmeal	2.7 oz	83	7	172
cracked-wheat bread	1 lb loaf	295	16	1,190
	0.9 oz slice	16	1	65
danish *See* DESSERTS: CAKES, PASTRIES, & PIES				
French bread	1 lb loaf	499	18	1,270
	1.2 oz slice	39	1	100

	Portion	Calcium (mg)	Total Fat (g)	Total Calor
fruit & nut quick bread, from mix	1.4 oz slice	12	2	118
honey wheatberry bread	1 oz slice	35	1	70
Italian bread	1 lb loaf	77	4	1,255
	1 oz slice	5	tr	85
matzo *See* CRACKERS				
mixed-grain bread	1 lb loaf	472	17	1,165
	0.9 oz slice	27	1	65
oatmeal bread	1 lb loaf	267	20	1,145
	0.9 oz slice	15	1	65
pita bread, white	1 piece (6½″ diam)	49	1	165
pumpernickel bread	1 lb loaf	322	16	1,160
	1.1 oz slice	23	1	80
raisin bread	1 lb loaf	463	18	1,260
	0.9 oz slice	25	1	65
roman meal bread	1 oz slice	31	1	68
rye bread, light	1 lb loaf	363	17	1,190
	0.9 oz slice	20	1	65
sourdough bread	1 oz slice	28	1	68
Vienna bread	1 lb loaf	499	18	1,270
	0.9 oz slice	28	1	70
wheat bread	1 lb loaf	572	19	1,160
	0.9 oz slice	32	1	65
wheatberry bread	1 oz slice	29	1	70
white bread	1 lb loaf	572	18	1,210
	0.9 oz slice	32	1	65
	0.7 oz slice	25	1	55
whole-wheat bread	1 lb loaf	327	20	1,110
	1 oz slice	20	1	70

Muffins

	Portion	Calcium (mg)	Total Fat (g)	Total Calor
blueberry				
from mix	1.6 oz	15	5	140
homemade	1.6 oz	54	5	135
bran				
from mix	1.6 oz	27	4	140
homemade	1.6 oz	60	6	125
corn				
from mix	1.6 oz	30	6	145
homemade	1.6 oz	66	5	145
English				
regular	2 oz	96	1	140
sourdough	2 oz	112	1	129

Rolls & Bagels

	Portion	Calcium (mg)	Total Fat (g)	Total Calor
bagel, plain or water, enriched	1 (3½″ diam)	32	2	200

	Portion	Calcium (mg)	Total Fat (g)	Total Calor
brown & serve roll	1	14	2	92
croissant	2 oz	20	12	235
dinner roll				
commercial	1 oz	14	2	85
homemade	1.2 oz	20	3	120
frankfurter or hamburger roll	1.4 oz	54	2	115
French roll, enriched	1.8 oz	8	tr	137
hard roll, commercial	1.2 oz	30	2	155
hoagie or submarine roll	4.8 oz	72	8	400
parkerhouse roll	0.6 oz	15	2	59
popover, homemade	1.8 oz	48	5	112
raisin roll	2.1 oz	45	2	165
rye roll	0.6 oz	6	2	55
dark, hard	1 oz	5	1	80
light, hard	1 oz	8	1	79
sandwich roll	1.8 oz	13	3	162
sesame seed roll	0.6 oz	15	2	59
sweet roll *See* DESSERTS: CAKES, PASTRIES, & PIES				
wheat roll	0.6 oz	6	2	52
white roll, homemade	1.2 oz	16	3	119
whole-wheat roll, homemade	1.2 oz	34	1	90

Tortillas

	Portion	Calcium (mg)	Total Fat (g)	Total Calor
taco/tostada shell, corn	0.4 oz	11	2	50
tortilla, corn	1.1 oz	42	1	65
canned	1.2 oz	?	1	75
tortilla, flour	1.1 oz	46	2	95

• BRAND NAME

Lender's Bagels

	Portion	Calcium (mg)	Total Fat (g)	Total Calor
plain, egg, poppy seed, or pumpernickel	1	20	1	150–160
garlic	1	<20	1	150–160
onion, sesame seed, or rye	1	40	0–1	150–160

Ortega

	Portion	Calcium (mg)	Total Fat (g)	Total Calor
taco/tostada shells	1	<20	2	50

Pepperidge Farm
BREADS

	Portion	Calcium (mg)	Total Fat (g)	Total Calor
cinnamon	2 slices	20	5	170
cracked-wheat	2 slices	20	2	140
Dijon rye	2 slices	40	2	160
Family pumpernickel	2 slices	40	2	160
honey bran	2 slices	20	2	190

	Portion	Calcium (mg)	Total Fat (g)	Total Calor
honey wheatberry	2 slices	20	2	140
multigrain, very thin	2 slices	20	1	80
oatmeal	2 slices	40	3	140
Party Dijon Slices	4 slices	20	1	70
Party Pumpernickel Slices	4 slices	20	1	70
Party Rye Slices	4 slices	20	1	60
raisin w/cinnamon	2 slices	20	3	150
Sandwich White	2 slices	40	2	130
seeded Family rye	2 slices	40	1	80
seedless rye	2 slices	40	2	160
Toasting White	2 slices	60	2	170
wheat	2 slices	20	3	190
wheat germ	2 slices	40	1	130
white	2 slices	40	3	145
white, very thin	2 slices	40	1	80
whole-wheat	2 slices	40	2	130
whole-wheat, very thin	2 slices	20	2	80

ENGLISH MUFFINS

plain	1	20	2	140
cinnamon raisin	1	40	2	150

OLD FASHIONED MUFFINS, FROZEN

blueberry	1	20	6	170
bran w/raisins	1	20	6	170
carrot walnut	1	40	6	200
chocolate chip	1	20	8	210
cinnamon swirl	1	20	6	190
corn	1	20	7	180

ROLLS

butter crescent	1	20	6	110
club, brown & serve	1	40	1	100
French style	1	40	1	110
golden twist	1	20	6	110
hamburger	1	40	2	130
onion sandwich buns w/ poppy seeds	1	40	3	150
parkerhouse	1	20	1	60
sourdough-style French	1	20	1	100

Pillsbury
BISCUITS

all	2	0	1–15	100–200

BREAD STICKS

soft	1	0	2	100

	Portion	Calcium (mg)	Total Fat (g)	Total Calor
DINNER ROLLS				
all	1	0	?	100–200
PIPIN' HOT DINNER ROLLS				
all	1″ slice	0	2	60–80

SWEET ROLLS & TURNOVERS See DESSERTS: CAKES, PASTRIES, & PIES

Sara Lee
BAGELS

plain	1	11	1	230
cinnamon & raisin	1	16	2	240
egg	1	14	2	240
onion	1	14	1	220
poppy seed	1	28	1	230

HEARTY FRUIT MUFFINS

apple cinnamon spice	1	27	8	220
banana nut bran	1	9	9	230
blueberry	1	24	8	200
oatmeal & fruit	1	31	9	230

L'ORIGINAL CROISSANTS

all butter	1	26	9	170
petite size	1	17	6	120
presliced	1	26	9	170
cheese	1	32	9	170
wheat & honey	1	28	9	170

LE PASTRIE CROISSANTS See DESSERTS: CAKES, PASTRIES, & PIES

LE SANDWICH CROISSANTS See ENTREES & MAIN COURSES, FROZEN

❏ BREAKFAST CEREALS, COLD & HOT

Cold Cereal

cornflakes, low-sodium	1 oz or about 1 c	12	tr	113
crisp rice, low-sodium	1 oz or about 1 c	19	tr	114

	Portion	Calcium (mg)	Total Fat (g)	Total Calor
granola, homemade	1 oz or about ¼ c	18	8	138
	1 c	76	33	595
oat flakes, fortified	1 oz or about ⅔ c	40	tr	105
	1 c	68	1	177
rice, puffed	½ oz or about 1 c	1	tr	57
wheat, puffed, plain	½ oz or about 1 c (heaping)	4	tr	52
wheat, shredded				
large biscuit	1 rectangular	10	tr	83
	2 round	15	1	133
small biscuit	1 oz or about ⅔ c	11	1	102
	⅞ oz box	9	1	89
wheat germ, toasted				
plain	1 oz or about ¼ c	13	3	108
	1 c	50	12	431
w/brown sugar & honey	1 oz or about ¼ c	9	2	107
	1 c	38	9	426

Hot Cereal

	Portion	Calcium (mg)	Total Fat (g)	Total Calor
corn grits				
regular & quick				
dry	1 c	3	2	579
	1 T	0	tr	36
cooked	1 c	1	1	146
	¾ c	1	tr	110
instant, prepared				
plain	1 pkt	7	tr	82
w/artificial cheese flavor	1 pkt	14	1	107
w/imitation bacon bits	1 pkt	6	1	104
w/imitation ham bits	1 pkt	7	tr	103
farina				
dry	1 c	25	1	649
	1 T	2	tr	40
cooked	1 c	4	tr	116
	¾ c	3	tr	87
grits; hominy grits See corn grits, above				
oatmeal See oats, below				
oats, regular, quick, & instant, nonfortified				
dry	⅓ c	14	2	104
cooked	1 c	20	2	145
	¾ c	15	2	108

	Portion	Calcium (mg)	Total Fat (g)	Total Calor

- **BRAND NAME**

Arrowhead Mills
COLD CEREAL

	Portion	Calcium (mg)	Total Fat (g)	Total Calor
Agrain & Agrain	2 oz	20	2	220
Arrowhead Crunch	1 oz	20	3	120
bran flakes	1 oz	<20	1	100
corn, puffed	½ oz	<20	0	50
cornflakes	1 oz	20	1	110
granola				
apple amaranth	2 oz	20	6	225
maple nut	2 oz	60	11	260
millet, puffed	½ oz	<20	0	50
Nature O's	1 oz	<20	1	110
rice, puffed	½ oz	<20	0	50
wheat, puffed	½ oz	<20	0	50
wheat bran	2 oz	60	2	200
wheat germ, raw	2 oz	40	6	210

HOT CEREAL

	Portion	Calcium (mg)	Total Fat (g)	Total Calor
Bear Mush	1 oz	<20	0	100
corn grits, white or yellow	2 oz	<20	1	200
4 Grain & Flax	2 oz	20	1	94
oat bran	1 oz	20	2	110
oatmeal, instant	1 oz	<20	2	100
oats, steel cut	2 oz	20	4	220
Rice & Shine	¼ c	20	1	160
Seven Grain	1 oz	20	1	100
wheat, cracked	2 oz	20	1	180

Erewhon
COLD CEREAL

	Portion	Calcium (mg)	Total Fat (g)	Total Calor
Crispy Brown Rice, regular or low-sodium	1 oz or about 1 c	3	1	110
Fruit 'n Wheat	1 oz or about ½ c	14	1	100
granola				
date nut	1 oz or about ¼ c	25	6	130
honey almond	1 oz or about ¼ c	16	6	130
maple	1 oz or about ¼ c	27	5	130
#9, w/bran, no salt added	1 oz or about ¼ c	24	6	130
spiced apple	1 oz or about ¼ c	30	6	130

	Portion	Calcium (mg)	Total Fat (g)	Total Calor
Sunflower Crunch	1 oz or about ¼ c	14	4	130
raisin bran	1 oz or about ½ c	tr	0	100
wheat flakes	1 oz or about ½ c	tr	0	110

HOT CEREAL

	Portion	Calcium (mg)	Total Fat (g)	Total Calor
Barley Plus	1 oz or about ⅓ c dry	2	1	110
brown rice cream	1 oz or about ⅓ c dry	11	1	110
oat bran w/toasted wheat germ	1 oz or about ⅓ c dry	17	2	115

General Mills Cold Cereal

	Portion	Calcium (mg)	Total Fat (g)	Total Calor
Cheerios regular	1 oz or about 1¼ c	48	2	111
	¾ oz box	36	1	83
Honey Nut	1 oz or about ¾ c	20	1	107
	1 c	23	1	125
Crispy Wheats 'n Raisins	1 oz or about ¾ c	47	1	99
	1 c	71	1	150
Golden Grahams	1 oz or about ¾ c	17	1	109
	1 c	24	2	150
Kix	1 oz or about 1½ c	35	1	110
	¾ oz box	27	1	83
Lucky Charms	1 oz or about 1 c	32	1	110
Total	1 oz or about 1 c	48	1	100
Trix	1 oz or about 1 c	6	tr	109
Wheaties	1 oz or about 1 c	43	1	99

Health Valley
COLD CEREAL

	Portion	Calcium (mg)	Total Fat (g)	Total Calor
Amaranth Crunch w/raisins	1 oz or about ¼ c	5	3	110
amaranth flakes	1 oz or about ½ c	20	1	110
amaranth w/banana	1 oz or about ¼ c	29	2	100
bran, w/apples & cinnamon or w/raisins	1 oz or about ¼ c	13	1	100

	Portion	Calcium (mg)	Total Fat (g)	Total Calor
Fiber 7 Flakes	1 oz or about ½ c	2	1	100
Fruit Lites				
corn	½ oz or about ½ c	3	0	43
rice	½ oz or about ½ c	5	0	45
wheat	½ oz or about ½ c	6	0	43
granola *See* Real Granola, *below*				
Healthy Crunch				
w/almonds & dates	1 oz or about ¼ c	17	3	120
w/apples & cinnamon	1 oz or about ¼ c	12	3	120
Lites				
corn	½ oz or about ½ c	3	0	50
rice	½ oz or about ½ c	5	0	50
wheat	½ oz or about ½ c	7	0	50
oat bran flakes				
plain	1 oz or about ½ c	17	2	110
w/almonds & dates	1 oz or about ½ c	20	2	110
w/raisins	1 oz or about ½ c	17	1	107
Orangeola				
w/almonds & dates	1 oz or about ¼ c	16	4	120
w/banana & Hawaiian fruit	1 oz or about ¼ c	14	4	120
raisin bran flakes	1 oz or about ½ c	13	0	110
Real Granola				
w/almond crunch or w/Hawaiian fruit	1 oz or about ¼ c	24	3	120
w/raisins & nuts	1 oz or about ¼ c	21	3	120
Sprouts 7				
w/bananas & Hawaiian fruit	1 oz or about ¼ c	15	1	100
w/raisins	1 oz or about ¼ c	13	1	100
stoned-wheat flakes	1 oz or about ⅔ c	13	0	110
Swiss Breakfast				
raisin nut	1 oz or about ¼ c	14	2	100

	Portion	Calcium (mg)	Total Fat (g)	Total Calor
tropical fruit	1 oz or about ¼ c	17	2	100
wheat bran/Millers Flakes	2 oz	68	3	121
wheat germ w/fiber, almonds & dates or bananas & tropical fruit	1 oz or about ¼ c	20	1	100

HOT CEREAL

hot oat bran w/apples	1 oz or ¼ c	16	1	110

Heartland Cold Cereal
Natural Cereal

	Portion	Calcium (mg)	Total Fat (g)	Total Calor
plain	1 oz or about ¼ c	19	4	123
	1 c	75	18	499
w/coconut	1 oz or about ¼ c	18	5	125
	1 c	67	17	463
w/raisins	1 oz or about ¼ c	17	4	120
	1 c	66	16	467

Kellogg's Cold Cereal

	Portion	Calcium (mg)	Total Fat (g)	Total Calor
All-Bran	1 oz or about ⅓ c	22	1	70
w/extra fiber	1 oz or about ½ c	28	1	60
w/fruit & almonds	1.3 oz or about ⅔ c	35	2	100
Apple Jacks	1 oz or about 1 c	3	0	110
Bran Buds	1 oz or about ⅓ c	20	1	70
bran flakes	1 oz or about ⅔ c	13	0	90
Cocoa Krispies	1 oz or about ¾ c	6	0	110
Corn Flakes				
regular	1 oz or about 1 c	1	0	110
honey & nut	1 oz or about ⅔ c	4	1	110
Corn Pops	1 oz or about 1 c	2	0	110
Cracklin' Oat Bran	1 oz or about ½ c	15	4	110
Crispix	1 oz or about 1 c	4	0	110
Froot Loops	1 oz or about 1 c	3	1	110
Frosted Flakes	1 oz or about ¾ c	1	0	110

	Portion	Calcium (mg)	Total Fat (g)	Total Calor
Frosted Krispies	1 oz or about ¾ c	2	0	110
Frosted Mini-Wheats	1 oz = about 4 biscuits	10	0	100
Fruitful Bran	1.3 oz or about ⅔ c	12	0	120
Honey Smacks	1 oz or about ¾ c	3	0	110
Just Right				
all-grain	1 oz or about ⅔ c	7	0	100
w/fruit	1.3 oz or about ¾ c	13	1	140
Nutri-Grain				
almond raisin	1.4 oz or about ⅔ c	16	2	150
corn	1 oz or about ½ c	1	1	100
wheat	1 oz or about ⅔ c	9	0	100
wheat & raisins	1.4 oz or about ⅔ c	13	0	130
Product 19	1 oz or about 1 c	4	0	110
raisin bran	1.4 oz or about ¾ c	19	1	120
Rice Krispies	1 oz or about 1 c	3	0	110
Special K	1 oz or about 1 c	10	0	110
Maltex Hot Cereal				
Maltex				
dry	¼ c	14	1	134
cooked	1 c	18	1	180
	¾ c	14	1	135
Old Fashioned Maltex	½ c cooked	7	tr	77
Malt-O-Meal Hot Cereal				
Malt-O-Meal, plain or chocolate				
dry	1 T	1	tr	38
cooked	1 c	5	tr	122
	¾ c	4	tr	92
Maypo				
Maypo				
dry	½ c	133	3	181
cooked	1 c	125	2	170
	¾ c	94	2	128
30-Second Oatmeal				
regular	½ c cooked	79	1	89
maple flavor	1 oz dry	80	1	101

	Portion	Calcium (mg)	Total Fat (g)	Total Calor
Vermont-Style Hot Oat Cereal	½ c cooked	59	1	77
Nabisco				
COLD CEREAL				
Fruit Wheats, apple, raisin, or strawberry	1 oz	<20	0	100
100% Bran	1 oz or about ½ c	20	1	76
	1 c	46	3	178
Shredded Wheat 'n Bran	1 oz	<20	1	110
Team	1 oz or about 1 c	4	1	111
Toasted Wheat & Raisins	1 oz	<20	1	100
HOT CEREAL				
Cream of Rice	1 oz dry	<20	0	100
Cream of Wheat				
instant	1 oz dry	150	0	100
regular	1 oz dry	40	0	100
Mix 'n Eat				
Original	1 oz dry	40	0	100
w/apple & cinnamon, w/ brown sugar cinnamon, or w/maple brown sugar	1¼ oz dry	40	0	130
w/peach or strawberry	1¼ oz dry	40	2	140
quick				
regular	1 oz dry	40	0	100
w/apples, raisins, & spice or w/maple brown sugar, artificially flavored	1 oz dry	40	1	110
Nature Valley Cold Cereal				
granola, toasted oat mixture	1 oz or about ⅓ c	18	5	126
	1 c	71	20	503
Post Cold Cereal				
Alpha-Bits	1 oz	<20	1	110
Cocoa Pebbles	1 oz	<20	1	110
C.W. Post Hearty Granola				
plain	1 oz	<20	4	130
w/raisins	1 oz	<20	4	120
Frosted Rice Krinkles	1 oz or about ⅞ c	4	tr	109
Fruit & Fibre: dates, raisins, walnuts; Harvest Medley; Mountain Trail; or tropical fruit	1 oz	<20	1	90
Fruity Pebbles	1 oz	<20	1	110
granola See C.W. Post Hearty Granola, *above*				
Grape-Nuts				
regular	1 oz	<20	0	110
raisin	1 oz	<20	0	100

	Portion	Calcium (mg)	Total Fat (g)	Total Calor
Grape-Nuts Flakes	1 oz	<20	1	100
Honeycomb	1 oz	<20	0	110
Natural Raisin Bran	1 oz	<20	0	80
oat flakes, fortified	1 oz	20	1	110
Post Toasties	1 oz	<20	0	110
Super Golden Crisp	1 oz or about ⅞ c	<20	0	110

Quaker Oats
COLD CEREAL

	Portion	Calcium (mg)	Total Fat (g)	Total Calor
bran, unprocessed	2 T	6	tr	21
Cap'n Crunch				
regular	1 oz or about ¾ c	5	3	119
	1 c	6	3	156
w/Crunchberries	1 oz or about ¾ c	9	2	118
	1 c	11	3	146
peanut butter	1 oz or about ¾ c	6	4	124
	1 c	7	5	154
corn bran	1 oz or about ⅔ c	33	1	98
	1 c	41	1	124
King Vitaman	1 oz or about 1¼ c	17	2	115
	1 c	13	1	85
100% Natural Cereal				
plain	1 oz or about ¼ c	49	6	133
	1 c	181	22	489
w/apples & cinnamon	1 oz or about ¼ c	43	5	130
	1 c	157	20	478
w/raisins & dates	1 oz or about ¼ c	41	5	128
	1 c	160	20	496
Life, plain or cinnamon	1 oz or about ⅔ c	99	1	104
	1 c	154	1	162
Mr. T	1 c	9	3	121
Quisp	1 oz or about 1 c	9	2	117

HOT CEREAL

	Portion	Calcium (mg)	Total Fat (g)	Total Calor
farina, quick creamy wheat	2½ T un-cooked	6	0	101
oat bran	⅓ c un-cooked	20	3	110
oats, instant, prepared				
regular	1 pkt	100	2	105

	Portion	Calcium (mg)	Total Fat (g)	Total Calor
w/apples & cinnamon	1 pkt	100	2	134
w/artificial maple & brown sugar	1 pkt	100	2	163
w/bran & raisins	1 pkt	100	2	153
w/cinnamon & spice	1 pkt	100	2	176
w/peaches & cream or w/ strawberries & cream, both artificially flavored	1 pkt	100	2	136
w/raisins & spice	1 pkt	100	2	159
w/raisins, dates, & walnuts	1 pkt	100	4	150
w/real honey & graham	1 pkt	100	2	136
Quaker Oats, Quick & Old Fashioned	⅓ c dry or ⅔ c cooked	14	2	109
Whole Wheat Hot Natural	⅓ c dry or ⅔ c cooked	9	1	106

Ralston Purina
COLD CEREAL

	Portion	Calcium (mg)	Total Fat (g)	Total Calor
Bran Chex	1 oz or about ⅔ c	17	1	91
	1 c	29	1	156
Cookie-Crisp	1 oz or about 1 c	5	1	114
Corn Chex	1 oz or about 1 c	3	tr	111
	¾ oz box	2	tr	84
cornflakes	1 oz or about 1 c	2	tr	111
raisin bran	1⅓ oz or about ¾ c	18	tr	120
	1 c	27	tr	178
Rice Chex	1 oz or about 1⅛ c	4	tr	112
	⅞ oz box	3	tr	98
sugar frosted flakes	1 oz or about ¾ c	3	tr	111
	1 c	4	1	149
Tasteeos	1 oz or about 1¼ c	13	1	111
	1 c	11	1	94
Wheat Chex	1 oz or about ⅔ c	11	1	104
	1 c	18	1	169

HOT CEREAL

Ralston

	Portion	Calcium (mg)	Total Fat (g)	Total Calor
dry	¼ c	11	1	102
cooked	1 c	14	1	134
	¾ c	10	1	100

	Portion	Calcium (mg)	Total Fat (g)	Total Calor
Roman Meal Hot Cereal				
Roman Meal				
plain				
dry	⅓ c	20	1	100
cooked	1 c	30	1	147
	¾ c	22	1	111
w/oats				
dry	¼ c	14	1	85
cooked	1 c	27	2	169
	¾ c	21	2	127
Sun Country Granola				
w/almonds	1 oz	23	5	130
w/raisins	1 oz	23	5	130
w/raisins & dates	1 oz	23	4	130
Sunshine				
shredded wheat				
regular	1 biscuit	<20	1	90
bite size	⅔ c	<20	1	110
U.S. Mills See also Erewhon, above				
Skinner's raisin bran	1 oz or about ½ c	?	1	100
Uncle Sam, laxative	1 oz or about ½ c	7	2	110
Wheatena Hot Cereal				
Wheatena				
dry	¼ c	10	1	125
cooked	1 c	11	1	135
	¾ c	8	1	101

❑ BREAKFAST FOODS, PREPARED

See also EGGS & EGG SUBSTITUTES; FAST FOODS

French toast, homemade	1 slice	72	7	155
pancakes				
from mix				
plain	1 (4″ diam)	36	2	60
buckwheat	1 (4″ diam)	59	2	55
homemade				
plain	1 (4″ diam)	27	2	60
cornmeal	1 (4″ diam)	23	1	68
soy	1 (4″ diam)	26	2	68
waffles				
from mix	1 (7″ diam)	179	8	205
frozen	1	28	3	95
homemade	1 (7″ diam)	154	13	245

	Portion	Calcium (mg)	Total Fat (g)	Total Calor
▪ BRAND NAME				
Arrowhead Mills Pancake Mixes				
Blue Heaven	½ c	150	2	200
buckwheat	½ c	250	2	270
Griddle Lite	½ c	200	3	260
multigrain	½ c	400	2	350
triticale	½ c	250	2	270
Aunt Jemima				
FRENCH TOAST, FROZEN				
plain	2 slices	94	4	168
cinnamon swirl	2 slices	94	6	190
raisin	2 slices	96	4	185
PANCAKE & WAFFLE MIXES				
original flavor	¼ c	140	1	108
buckwheat	¼ c	150	1	107
buttermilk	⅓ c	230	1	175
whole-wheat	⅓ c	181	1	142
PANCAKE BATTER, FROZEN				
original flavor	3 (4″ diam)	68	2	210
blueberry	3 (4″ diam)	68	2	205
buttermilk	3 (4″ diam)	91	2	212
PANCAKES, FROZEN				
original flavor	3 (4″ diam)	66	4	246
blueberry	3 (4″ diam)	67	4	249
buttermilk	3 (4″ diam)	76	4	240
WAFFLES, FROZEN				
original flavor	2	100	4	173
apple & cinnamon	2	100	4	173
blueberry	2	100	4	173
buttermilk	2	100	4	175
Fearn Pancake Mixes				
buckwheat	½ c dry	350	3	235
Rich Earth	½ c dry	300	2	190
7-grain buttermilk	½ c dry	350	2	200
stone-ground whole-wheat	½ c dry	350	2	220
unbleached wheat & soya	½ c dry	350	2	235
Health Valley				
7 Sprouted Grains buttermilk pancake & biscuit mix	1 oz	20	1	100

	Portion	Calcium (mg)	Total Fat (g)	Total Calor
Kellogg's				
EGGO FROZEN WAFFLES				
apple cinnamon	1	20	5	130
buttermilk	1	20	5	120
Homestyle	1	20	5	120
POP-TARTS See DESSERTS: CAKES, PASTRIES, & PIES				
Nabisco Toastettes *See* DESSERTS: CAKES, PASTRIES, & PIES				
Swanson				
GREAT STARTS BREAKFASTS				
French toast (cinnamon swirl)	6½ oz	100	28	480
French toast w/sausages	6½ oz	100	27	460
omelets w/cheese sauce & ham	7 oz	250	31	400
pancakes & blueberry sauce	7 oz	60	10	410
pancakes & sausages	6 oz	80	22	470
scrambled eggs & sausage w/ hashed brown potatoes	6¼ oz	60	34	430
Spanish-style omelet	7¾ oz	80	17	250
GREAT STARTS BREAKFAST SANDWICHES				
biscuit & sausage	4¾ oz	80	23	410
egg, Canadian bacon, & cheese/muffin	4½ oz	100	16	310
sausage, egg, & cheese/ biscuit	6¼ oz	200	32	520
steak, egg, & cheese/muffin	5¼ oz	100	23	390

❑ BROWNIES *See* COOKIES, BARS, & BROWNIES

❑ BUTTER & MARGARINE SPREADS

Butter

See also NUTS & NUT-BASED BUTTERS, FLOURS, MEALS, MILKS, PASTES, & POWDERS; SEEDS & SEED-BASED BUTTERS, FLOURS, & MEALS

	Portion	Calcium (mg)	Total Fat (g)	Total Calor
salted or unsalted	1 t	1	4	36
	1 stick = 4 oz or about ½ c	27	92	813
whipped, salted	1 t	1	3	27
	1 stick = 4 oz or about ½ c	18	61	542

	Portion	Calcium (mg)	Total Fat (g)	Total Calor

Margarine

REGULAR

Hard, Stick or Brick

	Portion	Calcium (mg)	Total Fat (g)	Total Calor
coconut, safflower, coconut (hydrogenated), & palm (hydrogenated)	1 stick	34	91	815
	1 t	1	4	34
corn (hydrogenated)	1 stick	34	91	815
	1 t	1	4	34
corn & corn (hydrogenated)	1 stick	34	91	815
	1 t	1	4	34
corn, soybean (hydrogenated), & cottonseed (hydrogenated)				
salted	1 stick	34	91	815
	1 t	1	4	34
unsalted	1 stick	20	91	810
	1 t	1	4	34
lard (hydrogenated)	1 stick	?	91	831
	1 t	?	4	35
safflower & soybean (hydrogenated)	1 stick	34	91	815
	1 t	1	4	34
safflower, soybean (hydrogenated), & cottonseed (hydrogenated)	1 stick	34	91	815
	1 t	1	4	34
safflower, soybean, soybean (hydrogenated), & cottonseed (hydrogenated)	1 stick	34	91	815
	1 t	1	4	34
soybean (hydrogenated)	1 stick	34	91	815
	1 t	1	4	34
soybean & soybean (hydrogenated)	1 stick	34	91	815
	1 t	1	4	34
soybean (hydrogenated) & cottonseed	1 stick	34	91	815
	1 t	1	4	34
soybean (hydrogenated) & cottonseed (hydrogenated)	1 stick	34	91	815
	1 t	1	4	34
soybean (hydrogenated) & palm (hydrogenated)	1 stick	34	91	815
	1 t	1	4	34
soybean (hydrogenated), corn, & cottonseed (hydrogenated)	1 stick	34	91	815
	1 t	1	4	34
soybean (hydrogenated), cottonseed (hydrogenated), & soybean	1 stick	34	91	815
	1 t	1	4	34
soybean (hydrogenated), palm (hydrogenated), & palm	1 stick	34	91	815
	1 t	1	4	34

	Portion	Calcium (mg)	Total Fat (g)	Total Calor
sunflower, soybean (hydrogenated), & cottonseed (hydrogenated)	1 stick 1 t	34 1	91 4	815 34
Liquid, Bottle				
soybean (hydrogenated), soybean, & cottonseed	1 c 1 t	150 3	183 4	1,637 34
Soft, Tub				
corn & corn (hydrogenated)	1 c 1 t	60 1	183 4	1,626 34
safflower, cottonseed (hydrogenated), & peanut (hydrogenated)	1 c 1 t	60 1	183 4	1,626 34
safflower & safflower (hydrogenated)	1 c 1 t	60 1	183 4	1,626 34
soybean (hydrogenated)				
salted	1 c 1 t	60 1	183 4	1,626 34
unsalted	1 c 1 t	60 1	182 4	1,626 34
soybean (hydrogenated) & cottonseed	1 c 1 t	60 1	183 4	1,626 34
soybean (hydrogenated) & cottonseed (hydrogenated)				
salted	1 c 1 t	60 1	183 4	1,626 34
unsalted	1 c 1 t	60 1	182 4	1,626 34
soybean (hydrogenated) & safflower	1 c 1 t	60 1	183 4	1,626 34
soybean (hydrogenated), cottonseed (hydrogenated), & soybean	1 c 1 t	60 1	183 4	1,626 34
soybean (hydrogenated), palm (hydrogenated), & palm	1 c 1 t	60 1	183 4	1,626 34
soybean, soybean (hydrogenated), & cottonseed (hydrogenated)	1 c 1 t	60 1	183 4	1,626 34
sunflower, cottonseed (hydrogenated), & peanut (hydrogenated)	1 c 1 t	60 1	183 4	1,626 34
IMITATION (ABOUT 40% FAT)				
corn & corn (hydrogenated)	1 c 1 t	41 1	90 2	801 17
soybean (hydrogenated)	1 c 1 t	41 1	90 2	801 17

	Portion	Calcium (mg)	Total Fat (g)	Total Calor
soybean (hydrogenated) & cottonseed	1 c	41	90	801
	1 t	1	2	17
soybean (hydrogenated) & cottonseed (hydrogenated)	1 c	41	90	801
	1 t	1	2	17
soybean (hydrogenated), palm (hydrogenated), & palm	1 c	41	90	801
	1 t	1	2	17
unspecified ingredient oils	1 c	41	90	801
	1 t	1	2	17

SPREAD, MARGARINELIKE (ABOUT 60% FAT)

Stick

	Portion	Calcium (mg)	Total Fat (g)	Total Calor
soybean (hydrogenated) & palm (hydrogenated)	1 c	48	139	1,236
	1 t	1	3	26

Tub

	Portion	Calcium (mg)	Total Fat (g)	Total Calor
soybean (hydrogenated) & cottonseed (hydrogenated)	1 c	48	139	1,236
	1 t	1	3	26
soybean (hydrogenated), palm (hydrogenated), & palm	1 c	48	139	1,236
	1 t	1	3	26
unspecified ingredient oils	1 c	48	139	1,236
	1 t	1	3	26

▪ BRAND NAME

Blue Bonnet Margarine

	Portion	Calcium (mg)	Total Fat (g)	Total Calor
Butter Blend, soft or stick, salted or unsalted	1 T	<20	11	90
margarine				
regular, soft or stick	1 T	<20	11	100
diet	1 T	<20	6	50
whipped, soft or stick	1 T	<20	7	70
spread				
Light Tasty, 52% vegetable oil	1 T	<20	7	60
52% fat	1 T	<20	8	80
stick, 70% fat	1 T	<20	10	90
stick, 75% fat	1 T	<20	11	90
whipped, 60% fat	1 T	<20	6	50

Fleischmann's

margarine

	Portion	Calcium (mg)	Total Fat (g)	Total Calor
regular: stick, soft, or squeeze; salted or un-salted	1 T	<20	11	100
diet or diet w/lite salt	1 T	<20	6	50
whipped, salted or unsalted	1 T	<20	7	70

	Portion	Calcium (mg)	Total Fat (g)	Total Calor
spread, light corn oil, soft or stick	1 T	<20	8	80
Land O'Lakes				
butter				
regular, salted or unsalted	1 T	<20	11	100
whipped, salted or unsalted	1 T	<20	7	60
Country Morning Blend margarine				
stick, salted or unsalted	1 T	<20	11	100
soft, tub, salted or unsalted	1 T	<20	10	90
margarine, stick or soft tub, regular (soy oil) or premium (corn oil)	1 T	<20	11	100
Mazola				
margarine				
regular, salted or unsalted	1 T	<20	11	100
diet	1 T	<20	6	50
Nucoa				
margarine	1 T	<20	11	100
soft margarine	1 T	<20	10	90

❏ **CAKES** *See* DESSERTS: CAKES, PASTRIES, & PIES

❏ **CANDIED FRUIT** *See* BAKING INGREDIENTS

❏ **CANDY**

butterscotch	6 pieces	6	3	116
butterscotch chips	1 oz	?	7	150
caramels				
plain or chocolate	3	41	3	112
plain or chocolate w/nuts	2	39	5	120
chocolate				
chocolate fudge center	1	30	5	129
chocolate fudge w/nuts center	1	28	6	127
coconut center	1	13	5	123
cream center	1	?	4	102
fondant center	1	16	3	115
vanilla cream center	1	34	4	114
chocolate chips				
chocolate-flavored	¼ c	13	8	195
dark	1 oz	8	8	148

	Portion	Calcium (mg)	Total Fat (g)	Total Calor
milk chocolate	¼ c	80	11	218
semisweet	1 c or 6 oz (60 chips/ oz)	51	61	860
chocolate-covered almonds	1 oz	57	12	159
chocolate-covered Brazil nuts	1 oz	57	14	162
chocolate-covered peanuts	1 oz	23	9	153
chocolate-covered raisins	1 oz	27	4	115
chocolate kisses	6	53	9	154
chocolate stars	7	64	8	145
English toffee	1 oz	0	17	193
fondant, uncoated (mints, candy corn, other)	1 oz	2	0	105
fudge				
chocolate, plain	1 oz	22	3	115
chocolate w/nuts	1 oz	22	5	119
vanilla	1 oz	31	3	111
vanilla w/nuts	1 oz	31	5	119
granola bars See COOKIES, BARS, & BROWNIES				
gum drops	1 oz	2	tr	100
hard candy	1 oz	tr	0	110
	6 pieces	6	tr	108
jelly beans	1 oz	1	tr	105
	10	3	0	66
lollipop	1 medium	0	0	108
malted milk balls	14	63	7	135
marshmallows	1 oz	1	0	90
	1 large	1	0	25
mints	14	2	1	104
peanut brittle	1 oz	11	4	123
sugar-coated almonds	7	28	5	128

▪ BRAND NAME

NOTE: Candies may be listed under product name (e.g., Milky Way) or company name (e.g., Cadbury or Hershey).

Almond Joy	1 oz	?	8	151
Baby Ruth	½ bar	<20	6	130
Baker's chocolate See BAKING INGREDIENTS				
Beechies candy-coated gum, all flavors	1 piece	<20	0	6
Beech-Nut				
cough drops, all flavors	1	<20	0	10
gum, all flavors	1 piece	<20	0	10
Bit-O-Honey	1 oz	13	4	121
	1.8 oz	24	7	220
Bonkers!, all flavors	1 piece	<20	0	20
Breath Savers Mints, sugar-free, all flavors	1	<20	0	8

	Portion	Calcium (mg)	Total Fat (g)	Total Calor
Bubble Yum bubble gum, all flavors				
regular	1 piece	<20	0	25
sugarless	1 piece	<20	0	20
Butterfinger	½ bar	<20	6	130
Butter Nut	1.8 oz	?	12	250
Cadbury				
chocolate almond	1 oz	?	9	155
chocolate Brazil nut	1 oz	?	9	156
chocolate hazelnut	1 oz	?	9	155
chocolate Krisp	1 oz	?	7	146
creme eggs	1 oz	?	6	136
fruit & nut	1 oz	?	9	152
milk chocolate	1 oz	?	8	151
Caramello	1 oz	?	8	144
Caravelle	1 oz	?	5	137
Care-Free				
sugarless bubble gum, all flavors	1 piece	<20	0	10
sugarless gum, all flavors	1 piece	<20	0	8
Charleston Chew!	½ piece	<20	3	120
Chunky				
Original	1 oz	35	7	143
milk chocolate	1 oz	51	4	120
peanut	1 oz	47	9	151
pecan	1 oz	33	8	148
Fruit Stripe				
bubble gum, all flavors	1 piece	<20	0	10
gum, all flavors	1 piece	<20	0	10
Good 'n Fruity	1½ oz	3	tr	160
Good & Plenty	1½ oz	69	tr	151
Hershey				
chocolate chips & unsweetened chocolate See BAKING INGREDIENTS				
chocolate Kisses	9 or 1.46 oz	80	13	220
Krackel	1.6 oz	80	14	250
milk chocolate	1.65 oz	80	14	250
milk chocolate w/almonds	1.55 oz	100	15	250
Special Dark sweet chocolate	1.45 oz	<20	12	220
Junior Mints	12	<20	3	120
Kit Kat	1.13 oz	48	9	162
	1.6 oz	100	13	250
Life Savers				
lollipops, all flavors	1	<20	0	45
milk chocolate stars	13	40	8	160
roll candy, all flavors, regular or sugar-free	1 piece	<20	0	8
M&M's				
regular	1.59 oz	?	10	220
peanut	1.67 oz	?	12	240
Marathon	1.38 oz	?	7	179

	Portion	Calcium (mg)	Total Fat (g)	Total Calor
Mars	1.7 oz	?	10	230
Milk Mounds	1 oz	?	8	138
Milk Shake	2 oz	?	8	250
Milky Way	2.1 oz	?	9	260
Mounds	1 oz	?	7	147
Mr. Goodbar	1.27 oz	50	12	198
	1.85 oz	60	20	300
Mr. Goodbar, big block	2 oz	79	18	300
Nestlé				
Crunch	1.06 oz	?	8	160
milk chocolate	1.07 oz	?	9	160
milk chocolate w/almonds	1 oz	?	9	150
Oh Henry!	1 oz	19	7	139
	2 oz	38	14	278
Pay Day	1.9 oz	?	12	250
Pearson's				
Carmel Nip	4	20	3	120
Coffee Nip	4	20	3	120
Licorice Nip	4	20	3	120
Chocolate Parfait	4	20	3	120
Peppermint Pattie	1 oz	?	2	124
Pillsbury food sticks	4	?	6	180
Planters				
peanut bar				
regular	1.6 oz	<20	11	230
honey roasted	1.6 oz	<20	13	230
Sweet 'n Crunchy	1.6 oz	<20	15	250
Old Fashioned peanut candy	1 oz	<20	9	140
Pom Poms	½ box	20	3	100
Power House	1 oz	?	5	131
Reese's				
Peanut Butter Cup	1.8 oz	20	17	280
peanut butter–flavored chips	¼ c	46	13	223
Pieces	1.95 oz	40	11	270
Rolo	9 pieces or 1.95 oz	60	12	270
Skor	1.4 oz	20	14	220
Snickers	2 oz	?	13	270
Sno-Caps	1 oz	7	4	132
Starbar	1 oz	?	7	141
Sugar Babies	1 pkg	20	2	180
Sugar Daddy	1	20	1	150
Summit	0.76 oz	?	6	100
Thousand Dollar	1½ oz	?	8	200
Three Musketeers	2.28 oz	?	8	280
Twix	1.73 oz	?	6	120
Whatchamacallit	1.8 oz	20	15	270
Y&S Bites or Twizzlers	1 oz	<20	<1	100
Zero	2 oz	45	8	250

	Portion	Calcium (mg)	Total Fat (g)	Total Calor

❑ **CANNED MEATS** *See* PROCESSED MEAT & POULTRY PRODUCTS

❑ **CEREAL, BREAKFAST** *See* BREAKFAST CEREALS, COLD & HOT

❑ **CHEESE & CHEESE FOODS**

Natural Cheese

	Portion	Calcium (mg)	Total Fat (g)	Total Calor
bleu	1 oz	150	8	100
	1 c, crumbled, not packed	712	39	477
brick	1" cube	116	5	64
	1 oz	191	8	105
Brie	1 oz	52	8	95
	4½ oz	236	35	427
Camembert	1 oz	110	7	85
	3⅓ oz	147	9	114
caraway	1 oz	191	8	107
cheddar	1 oz	204	9	114
	1 c, shredded, not packed	815	37	455
Cheshire	1 oz	182	9	110
Colby	1" cube	118	6	68
	1 oz	194	9	112
cottage				
creamed, small curd	4 oz	68	5	117
	1 c, not packed	126	9	217
fruit added	4 oz	54	4	140
	1 c, not packed	108	8	279
dry curd	4 oz	36	tr	96
	1 c, not packed	46	tr	123
low-fat				
2%	4 oz	77	2	101
	1 c, not packed	155	4	203
1%	4 oz	69	1	82
	1 c, not packed	138	2	164
cream	1 oz	23	10	99
	3 oz	68	30	297

	Portion	Calcium (mg)	Total Fat (g)	Total Calor
Edam	1 oz	207	8	101
	7 oz	1,447	55	706
feta, from sheep's milk	1 oz	140	6	75
fontina	1 oz	156	9	110
	8 oz	1,248	71	883
gjetost, from goats' & cows'	1 oz	113	8	132
milk	8 oz	908	67	1,057
Gouda	1 oz	198	8	101
	7 oz	1,386	54	705
Gruyère	1 oz	287	9	117
	6 oz	1,719	55	702
Limburger	1 oz	141	8	93
	8 oz	1,128	62	742
Monterey Jack	1 oz	212	9	106
	6 oz	1,269	51	635
mozzarella	1 oz	147	6	80
low-moisture	1″ cube	101	4	56
	1 oz	163	7	90
part skim	1″ cube	129	3	49
	1 oz	207	5	79
part skim	1 oz	183	5	72
Muenster	1 oz	203	9	104
	6 oz	1,219	51	626
Neufchâtel	1 oz	21	7	74
	3 oz	64	20	221
Parmesan				
grated	1 T	69	2	23
	1 oz	390	9	129
hard	1 oz	336	7	111
	5 oz	1,681	37	557
Port du Salut	1 oz	184	8	100
	6 oz	1,105	48	598
provolone	1 oz	214	8	100
	6 oz	1,285	45	598
ricotta				
whole milk	½ c	257	16	216
part skim milk	½ c	337	10	171
Romano, hard	1 oz	302	8	110
	5 oz	1,511	38	549
Roquefort, from sheep's milk	1 oz	188	9	105
	3 oz	563	26	314
Swiss	1″ cube	144	4	56
	1 oz	272	8	107
Tilsit	1 oz	198	7	96
	6 oz	1,190	44	578

whey *See* MILK, MILK SUBSTITUTES, & MILK PRODUCTS

	Portion	Calcium (mg)	Total Fat (g)	Total Calor

Process Cheese & Cheese Food

CHEESE FOOD

American
cold pack	1 oz	141	7	94
	8 oz	1,129	56	752
pasteurized process	1 oz	163	7	93
	8 oz	1,303	56	745
Swiss, pasteurized process	1 oz	205	7	92
	8 oz	1,642	55	734

CHEESE SPREAD

American, pasteurized process	1 oz	159	6	82
	5 oz	798	30	412

PASTEURIZED PROCESS CHEESE

American	1" cube	108	5	66
	1 oz	174	9	106
pimiento	1" cube	108	5	66
	1 oz	174	9	106
Swiss	1" cube	138	4	60
	1 oz	219	7	95

• BRAND NAME

Armour
cheddar, regular or lower salt	1 oz	200	9	110
Colby, regular or lower salt	1 oz	200	9	110
Monterey Jack, regular or lower salt	1 oz	200	9	110

Bonbel *See* Fromageries Bel, *below*
Delicia Pasteurized Process Cheese Substitute
American	1 oz	233	6	80
American w/peppers	1 oz	215	6	80
Hickory Smoked American	1 oz	237	6	80

Friendship
cottage cheese
California style, 4% milk fat	½ c	60	5	120
Friendship 'n Fruit	6 oz	80	1	100
low-fat				
regular or lactose-reduced, both 1% milk fat	½ c	60	1	90
large curd pot style, 2% milk fat	½ c	60	2	100
w/pineapple, 4% milk fat	½ c	60	4	140
cream cheese	1 oz	20	<10	103
farmer cheese	½ c	120	12	160
natural hoop cheese, ½% milk fat	4 oz	20	<1	84

	Portion	Calcium (mg)	Total Fat (g)	Total Calor
Fromageries Bel				
Babybel	1 oz	199	7	91
Bombino	1 oz	204	9	103
Bonbel	1 oz	182	8	100
cheddar	1 oz	212	9	110
Edam	1 oz	197	8	100
Gouda	1 oz	212	9	110
Mini Babybel	¾ oz	137	6	74
Mini Bonbel	¾ oz	137	6	74
Mini Gouda	¾ oz	160	6	80
Reduced Mini	¾ oz	157	3	45
Hoffman's				
CHEESE FOOD				
American	1 oz	146	7	100
Chees'n Bacon	1 oz	132	6	90
Chees'n Onion	1 oz	148	7	100
Chees'n Salami	1 oz	140	6	90
Hot Pepper w/jalapeño peppers	1 oz	150	7	90
Swisson Rye w/caraway	1 oz	151	7	90
PASTEURIZED PROCESS CHEESE				
American	1 oz	146	9	110
cheddar				
Smokey Sharp	1 oz	136	9	110
Super Sharp	1 oz	146	8	110
Smokey Swiss'n Cheddar	1 oz	170	8	110
Land O'Lakes				
CULTURED CHEESE				
cottage cheese	4 oz	60	5	120
cottage cheese, 2% milk fat	4 oz	80	2	100
NATURAL CHEESE				
brick	1 oz	200	8	110
cheddar	1 oz	200	9	110
Colby	1 oz	200	9	110
Edam	1 oz	200	8	100
Gouda	1 oz	200	8	100
Monterey Jack	1 oz	200	9	110
mozzarella, low-moisture, part skim	1 oz	200	5	80
Muenster	1 oz	200	9	100
provolone	1 oz	200	8	100
Swiss	1 oz	250	8	110
PROCESS CHEESE & CHEESE FOOD				
American	1 oz	150	9	110
Golden Velvet cheese spread	1 oz	150	6	80
jalapeño cheese food	1 oz	150	7	90

	Portion	Calcium (mg)	Total Fat (g)	Total Calor
onion cheese food	1 oz	200	7	90
pepperoni cheese food	1 oz	150	7	90
Laughing Cow				
average values of cheese spreads	1 oz	150	6	78
May-Bud				
Edam	1 oz	207	8	100
farmers, semisoft, part skim	1 oz	150	7	90
Gouda	1 oz	198	8	100
Monterey Jack	1 oz	212	9	110
Nabisco Easy Cheese				
pasteurized process cheese spread, all flavors	1 oz	100	6	80
Wispride Cold Pack Cheese Food				
port wine	1 oz	150	7	100
sharp cheddar	1 oz	150	7	100

❏ CHICKEN *See* POULTRY, FRESH & PROCESSED

❏ CHUTNEYS *See* PICKLES, OLIVES, RELISHES, & CHUTNEYS

❏ COATINGS, SEASONED *See* BREADCRUMBS, CROUTONS, STUFFINGS, & SEASONED COATINGS

❏ CONDIMENTS *See* SAUCES, GRAVIES, & CONDIMENTS

❏ COOKIES, BARS, & BROWNIES

animal cookies	15	3	3	120
arrowroot cookies	2	6	2	47
brownies				
butterscotch	1 oz	31	5	115
chocolate, w/nuts				
commercial, frosted	0.9 oz	13	4	100
homemade, w/vegetable oil	0.7 oz	9	6	95
cherry coolers	2	3	2	58

	Portion	Calcium (mg)	Total Fat (g)	Total Calor
chocolate chip cookies				
commercial	4 (2¼″ diam)	13	9	180
from refrigerator dough	4 (2¼″ diam)	13	11	225
homemade, w/vegetable shortening	4 (2⅓″ diam)	13	11	185
w/coconut	1	8	4	82
chocolate cookies	1	11	3	93
chocolate sandwich cookies	1	3	2	49
chocolate snaps	4	5	2	53
coconut bars	1	16	5	109
fig bars	4 = 2 oz	40	4	210
	1	10	1	53
gingersnaps				
commercial	3 small	9	1	50
homemade	1	3	2	34
golden fruit cookies	1	13	1	63
graham crackers	2	6	1	60
chocolate-covered	1	15	3	62
granola bars	1	14	4	109
lemon coolers	2	4	2	57
macaroons	1	4	3	67
molasses cookies	1	15	3	71
oatmeal cookies, homemade	1	11	3	62
oatmeal raisin cookies				
from refrigerator dough	1	4	3	61
homemade	4 (2⅝″ diam)	18	10	245
peanut butter bars	1	28	10	198
peanut butter cookies				
from refrigerator dough	1	12	3	50
homemade	4 = 1.7 oz	21	14	245
peanut cookies	1	5	2	57
sandwich-type cookies, chocolate or vanilla	4 = 1.4 oz	12	8	195
shortbread cookies				
commercial	4 small	13	8	155
homemade, w/margarine	2 large	6	8	145
social tea cookies	2	2	1	43
sugar cookies				
from refrigerator dough	4 = 1.7 oz	50	12	235
homemade	1	16	3	89
sugar wafers	2	4	2	53
vanilla cream sandwich cookies	1	4	3	69
vanilla wafers	10 = 1.4 oz	16	7	185
Vienna finger sandwich cookies	1	6	3	72

	Portion	Calcium (mg)	Total Fat (g)	Total Calor
■ BRAND NAME				
Health Valley				
Animal Snaps				
cinnamon	6	7	1	15
vanilla	6	2	1	15
fruit bars, apple, date, or raisin	2	20	4	180
Fruit Jumbos				
almonds & dates or raisins & nuts	1	8	3	85
oat bran	1	?	3	80
tropical fruit	1	10	3	85
graham crackers				
amaranth	3	13	1	50
oat bran	3	9	2	54
Jumbos				
amaranth	1	20	2	60
cinnamon	1	20	2	70
oatmeal	1	17	2	60
peanut butter	1	20	2	70
tofu cookies	4	6	3	52
wheat-free cookies	4	5	3	52
Hershey New Trail Granola Snack Bars				
chocolate chip	1	<20	9	190
chocolate-covered cocoa creme	1	40	12	200
chocolate-covered honey graham	1	20	12	200
chocolate-covered peanut butter	1	40	11	200
peanut butter	1	20	9	190
peanut butter & chocolate chip	1	<20	9	180
Kellogg's Rice Krispies Bars				
chocolate chip	1	6	4	120
Cocoa Krispies chocolate chip	1	6	4	120
raisin	1	7	2	120
Nabisco				
Almost Home Family-Style cookies				
fudge chocolate chip cookies	2	<20	5	130
fudge & nut brownies	1	<20	7	160
fudge & vanilla creme sandwiches	1	20	6	140
iced Dutch apple fruit sticks	1	<20	1	70
oatmeal raisin cookies	2	<20	5	130
peanut butter chocolate chip cookies	2	<20	6	140

	Portion	Calcium (mg)	Total Fat (g)	Total Calor
Real chocolate chip cookies	2	<20	5	130
Old Fashioned sugar cookies	2	20	5	130
Apple Newtons	1	<20	2	110
Barnum's Animals (animal crackers)	11	<20	4	130
Bugs Bunny graham cookies	9	20	4	120
Cameo creme sandwiches	2	<20	5	140
Chewy Chips Ahoy!	2	<20	6	130
Chips 'n More	2	<20	7	150
chocolate grahams	3	<20	7	150
chocolate snaps	7	<20	4	130
Cinnamon Treats	2	<20	1	60
Cookies 'n Fudge	3	<20	8	150
devil's food cakes	1	<20	1	110
Famous chocolate wafers	5	<20	4	130
Giggles vanilla sandwich cookies	2	<20	6	140
graham or Honey Maid graham crackers	2	<20	1	60
imported Danish cookies	5	20	8	150
I Screams n' You Screams Double Dip chocolate creme sandwiches	2	<20	7	150
Lorna Doone shortbread	4	<20	7	140
Mallomars	2	<20	6	130
National arrowroot biscuits	6	20	4	130
Old Fashion ginger snaps	4	20	3	120
Oreo chocolate sandwich cookies	3	<20	6	140
Oreo mint creme chocolate sandwich cookies	2	<20	6	150
Pantry molasses cookies	2	20	4	130
pecan shortbread cookies	2	<20	9	150
Pinwheels	1	<20	5	130
Social Tea biscuits	6	<20	4	130

Pepperidge Farm
ASSORTMENT COOKIES

Champagne	2	<20	6	110
Original Pirouettes	2	<20	6	110
Seville	2	<20	5	100

DISTINCTIVE COOKIES

Bordeaux	3	20	5	110
Brussels	3	<20	9	170
Chessmen	3	<20	6	130
Geneva	3	<20	11	190
Lido	2	20	11	180
Milano	3	<20	7	130

	Portion	Calcium (mg)	Total Fat (g)	Total Calor
Nassau	2	20	10	170
Orleans	3	<20	5	100
FRUIT COOKIES				
apricot-raspberry	3	<20	6	150
KITCHEN HEARTH COOKIES				
date nut granola	3	20	8	170
raisin bran	3	<20	8	160
OLD FASHIONED COOKIES				
brownie chocolate nut	3	20	10	170
chocolate chip	3	20	7	150
chocolate chocolate chip	3	20	8	160
Gingerman	3	20	4	100
hazelnut	3	<20	8	170
Irish oatmeal	3	<20	6	150
Lemon Nut Crunch	3	20	10	180
Molasses Crisps	3	20	4	100
oatmeal raisin	3	20	7	170
shortbread	3	<20	7	130
sugar	3	<20	7	150
SPECIAL COLLECTION COOKIES				
Almond Supreme	2	20	10	140
Chocolate Chunk Pecan	2	<20	7	130
milk chocolate macadamia	2	<20	8	140
Quaker Oats				
CHEWY GRANOLA BARS				
chocolate chip	1	26	5	129
chocolate, graham, & marsh-mallow	1	25	4	126
chunky nut & raisin	1	24	6	133
honey & oats	1	28	4	125
peanut butter	1	26	5	130
raisin & cinnamon	1	28	5	130
GRANOLA DIPPS BARS				
chocolate chip	1	29	6	138
honey & oats	1	30	6	137
peanut butter	1	23	7	141
raisin & almond	1	26	6	139
Sunshine				
animal crackers	14	<20	3	120
butter-flavored cookies	4	<20	5	120
Chip-A-Roos	2	<20	7	130
Chips'n Middles	2	<20	6	140
chocolate fudge sandwiches	2	<20	7	150

	Portion	Calcium (mg)	Total Fat (g)	Total Calor
cinnamon graham crackers	4, after breaking	<20	3	70
Country Style oatmeal cookies	2	<20	5	110
fig bars	2	20	2	90
ginger snaps	5	<20	3	100
Golden Fruit raisin biscuits	2, after breaking	<20	3	150
honey graham crackers	4, after breaking	<20	2	60
Hydrox	3	<20	7	160
Mallopuffs	2	<20	4	140
sugar wafers	3	<20	6	130
vanilla wafers	6	<20	6	130
Vienna fingers	2	<20	6	140

❑ CORNMEAL See FLOURS & CORNMEALS

❑ CRACKERS
See also SNACKS

bread sticks See BREADS, ROLLS, BISCUITS, & MUFFINS				
cheese, plain	10 (1" square)	11	3	50
cheese & peanut butter sandwich	1	7	2	40
graham See COOKIES, BARS, & BROWNIES				
matzo	1	?	tr	117
melba toast, plain	1	6	tr	20
oyster	33	4	3	120
rusk	1	2	1	42
rye crisp	2 triple crackers	5	tr	50
rye wafers, whole-grain	2 = ½ oz	7	1	55
saltines	4	3	1	50
snack-type cracker, standard, round	1	3	1	15
soda, unsalted tops	10	4	3	120
taco shells See BREADS, ROLLS, BISCUITS, & MUFFINS				
tortillas See BREADS, ROLLS, BISCUITS, & MUFFINS				
wheat, thin	4	3	1	35
whole-wheat wafers	2	3	2	35
zwieback See INFANT & TODDLER FOODS				

	Portion	Calcium (mg)	Total Fat (g)	Total Calor
■ BRAND NAME				
Cracottes				
regular or salt-free	1	<20	tr	12
whole-wheat	1	<20	tr	13
Health Valley				
Cheese Wheels	12	41	7	140
French onion, regular or no salt	13	40	6	130
herb				
regular	13	16	6	130
no salt	13	12	6	130
honey graham	13	11	6	130
sesame				
regular	13	31	6	130
no salt	13	27	6	130
7-Grain Vegetable				
regular	1 oz	17	6	130
no salt	1 oz	1	5	120
stoned-wheat				
regular	13	14	6	130
no salt	13	9	6	130
Nabisco				
Bacon-Flavored Thins	7	<20	4	70
Better Blue Cheese	10	<20	4	70
Better Cheddars	11	<20	4	70
Better Cheddars 'n' Bacon	10	<20	4	70
Better Nacho	9	<20	4	70
Better Swiss Cheese	10	<20	4	70
cheese peanut butter sandwich	2	20	3	70
Cheese Tid-Bits	16	20	4	70
Cheese Wheat Thins	9	20	3	70
Chicken in a Biskit	7	<20	4	70
Crown Pilot	1	<20	1	60
Dandy Soup & Oyster	20	<20	1	60
Dip in a Chip Cheese 'n Chive	8	20	4	70
Escort	3	<20	4	80
graham or Honey Maid graham crackers *See* COOKIES, BARS, & BROWNIES				
Great Crisps! *See* SNACKS				
Holland Rusk	1	<20	1	60
Meal Mates	3	20	3	70
Nips *See* SNACKS				
Nutty Wheat Thins	7	<20	5	80
Oysterettes	18	<20	1	60
Premium saltines, regular or low-salt	5	20	2	60
Ritz				
regular or low-salt	4	20	4	70
cheese	5	20	3	70

	Portion	Calcium (mg)	Total Fat (g)	Total Calor
Royal Lunch Milk	1	20	2	60
Sea Rounds	1	<20	2	60
Sociables	6	20	3	70
Toasted Peanut Butter Sandwich	2	<20	4	70
Triscuits, regular or low-salt	3	<20	2	60
Twigs, sesame or cheese	5	40	4	70
Uneeda Biscuit, unsalted tops	3	<20	2	60
Vegetable Thins	7	40	4	70
Waverly	4	20	3	70
Wheatsworth	5	<20	3	70
Wheat Thins, regular or low-salt	8	<20	3	70
Pepperidge Farm				
butter-flavored thin crackers	4	<20	3	80
English water biscuits	4	<20	1	70
Hearty wheat crackers	4	<20	4	100
sesame crackers	4	<20	3	80
Snack Sticks *See* SNACKS				
three-cracker assortment	4	<20	4	100
Tiny Goldfish *See* SNACKS				
Pillsbury				
bread sticks *See* BREADS, ROLLS, BISCUITS, & MUFFINS				
Quaker Oats				
rice cakes, lightly salted				
plain	1	2	tr	35
multigrain	1	3	tr	35
sesame	1	1	tr	35
Sunshine				
American Heritage				
cheddar	5	20	4	80
sesame	4	<20	4	70
Cheez-It	12	20	4	70
Hi Ho	4	<20	5	80
Krispy saltines	5	<20	1	60
oyster & soup	16	<20	2	60
wheat wafers	8	<20	4	80

❑ **CREAM & CREAM SUBSTITUTES**
See MILK, MILK SUBSTITUTES,
& MILK PRODUCTS

❑ **CROUTONS** *See* BREADCRUMBS,
CROUTONS, STUFFINGS,
& SEASONED COATINGS

	Portion	Calcium (mg)	Total Fat (g)	Total Calor

❏ **CUSTARDS** *See* DESSERTS: CUSTARDS, GELATINS, PUDDINGS, & PIE FILLINGS

❏ **DELI MEATS** *See* PROCESSED MEAT & POULTRY PRODUCTS

❏ **DESSERTS: CAKES, PASTRIES, & PIES**

Cake & Coffee Cake

	Portion	Calcium (mg)	Total Fat (g)	Total Calor
angel food				
from mix	whole (9¾" diam tube)	527	2	1,510
	¹⁄₁₂ cake	44	tr	125
homemade	2.1 oz	7	tr	161
banana, w/buttercream icing	1.8 oz	32	7	181
Boston cream pie	3.9 oz	74	10	332
caramel, from mix	1.6 oz	35	8	173
w/caramel icing	1.9 oz	46	8	208
carrot, w/cream cheese icing, homemade	whole (10" diam tube)	707	328	6,175
	¹⁄₁₆ cake	44	21	385
cheesecake				
commercial	whole (9" diam)	622	213	3,350
	¹⁄₁₂ cake	52	18	280
from mix	⅛ cake	181	14	300
chocolate, w/icing, from mix	1.3 oz cup-cake	47	5	129
coffee cake, crumb, from mix	whole (15.1 oz)	262	41	1,385
	⅙ cake	44	7	230
cottage pudding, homemade	1.8 oz	45	6	172
w/chocolate sauce	2½ oz	50	6	223
w/fruit sauce	2½ oz	51	6	204
devil's food, homemade	2.1 oz	68	11	227
devil's food, w/chocolate icing				
from mix, made w/margarine	whole, 2-layer (8" or 9" diam)	653	136	3,755
	¹⁄₁₆ cake	41	8	235
	1.2 oz cup-cake	21	4	120
homemade	2.1 oz	50	11	233

	Portion	Calcium (mg)	Total Fat (g)	Total Calor
fruitcake				
dark, homemade	3 lbs	1,293	228	5,185
	1½ oz	41	7	165
light	1.4 oz	27	7	156
gingerbread				
from mix	whole (8" square)	513	39	1,575
	⅑ cake	57	4	175
homemade	2½ oz	48	13	267
marble, w/white icing, from mix	1.8 oz	39	4	165
marble streusel, w/icing, from mix	2.3 oz	34	10	224
orange, w/icing, homemade	1.8 oz	37	7	183
pineapple upside-down, homemade	2.6 oz	54	9	236
pound				
commercial	1.1 lb loaf	146	94	1,935
	1 oz	8	5	110
homemade	1.1 lb loaf	339	94	2,025
	1 oz	20	5	120
sheet, plain, homemade, w/ vegetable oil				
unfrosted	whole (9" square)	495	108	2,830
	⅑ cake	55	12	315
w/uncooked white icing	whole (9" square)	548	129	4,020
	⅑ cake	61	14	445
shortcake	0.9 oz	10	2	86
w/blackberries	5.2 oz	105	8	347
w/peaches	5.3 oz	31	6	266
w/raspberries	5.6 oz	72	7	290
w/strawberries	6.2 oz	73	9	344
snack cake, small, commercial				
devil's food w/cream filling	1 oz	21	4	105
sponge w/cream filling	1½ oz	14	5	155
spice, from mix	1.8 oz	31	6	175
w/vanilla icing	1.8 oz	35	5	176
sponge, homemade	2.3 oz	25	3	188
w/strawberries & whipped cream	5.4 oz	45	8	328
white				
from mix	2½ oz	34	10	219
homemade	2.7 oz	87	12	285
white, w/chocolate icing, homemade	2.7 oz	62	12	298
white, w/white icing, commercial	whole, 2-layer (8" or 9" diam)	536	148	4,170
	1/16 cake	33	9	260

	Portion	Calcium (mg)	Total Fat (g)	Total Calor
yellow, homemade	2.6 oz	89	12	283
yellow, w/chocolate icing				
commercial	whole, 2-layer (8″ or 9″ diam)	366	175	3,895
	¹⁄₁₆ cake	23	11	245
from mix	whole, 2-layer (8″ or 9″ diam)	1,008	125	3,735
	¹⁄₁₆ cake	63	8	235
yellow, w/vanilla icing	1.4 oz cup-cake	16	6	160

Cake Icing

caramel	1.4 oz	39	5	140
chocolate	1.4 oz	23	6	148
chocolate fudge	1.4 oz	8	4	150
coconut	1.4 oz	4	3	140
white, fluffy	0.6 oz	4	0	70

Danish, Doughnuts, Sweet Rolls, & Toaster Pastries

danish pastry				
plain, w/out fruit or nuts	12 oz ring	360	71	1,305
	1 (4¼″ diam)	60	12	220
	1 oz	30	6	110
fruit	1 round	17	13	235
doughnut				
cake type, plain	1.8 oz	22	12	210
yeast-leavened, glazed	2.1 oz	17	13	235
sweet roll	1	11	7	154
toaster pastries	1	104	6	210

Fruit Bettys, Cobblers, Crisps, & Turnovers

apple brown Betty	½ c	25	5	211
apple crisp	½ c	10	8	302
apple dumpling	1	1	17	280
cherry crisp	½ c	26	tr	226
peach cobbler	⅓ c	7	6	160
peach crisp	½ c	10	9	249

Pastry

cream puff w/custard filling	3.7 oz	85	15	245
éclair				
w/chocolate icing & custard filling	3.9 oz	90	15	316

	Portion	Calcium (mg)	Total Fat (g)	Total Calor
frozen	2 oz	10	10	205
w/chocolate icing & whipped cream filling	3.7 oz	48	26	296
lady finger, w/whipped cream filling	4 oz	52	17	326
pastry shells & pie crusts *See* BAKING INGREDIENTS				

Pie

	Portion	Calcium (mg)	Total Fat (g)	Total Calor
apple, w/vegetable shortening crust	whole (9″ diam)	76	105	2,420
	⅙ pie	13	18	405
banana custard, homemade	5.6 oz	106	15	353
blackberry, homemade	5.6 oz	30	18	389
blueberry, w/vegetable shortening crust	whole (9″ diam)	104	102	2,285
	⅙ pie	17	17	380
butterscotch, homemade	5.6 oz	120	18	427
cherry, w/vegetable shortening crust	whole (9″ diam)	132	107	2,465
	⅙ pie	22	18	410
chocolate chiffon, homemade	2.8 oz	19	12	262
chocolate cream, homemade	4 oz	96	17	301
coconut custard, homemade	5½ oz	145	19	365
cream, w/vegetable shortening crust	whole (9″ diam)	273	139	2,710
	⅙ pie	46	23	455
custard, w/vegetable shortening crust	whole (9″ diam)	874	101	1,985
	⅙ pie	146	17	330
fried				
apple	3 oz	12	14	255
cherry	3 oz	11	14	250
lemon chiffon, homemade	3.8 oz	23	10	288
lemon meringue, w/vegetable shortening crust	whole (9″ diam)	118	86	2,140
	⅙ pie	20	14	355
mincemeat, homemade	5.6 oz	45	18	434
peach, w/vegetable shortening crust	whole (9″ diam)	95	101	2,410
	⅙ pie	16	17	405
pecan, w/vegetable shortening crust	whole (9″ diam)	388	189	3,450
	⅙ pie	65	32	575
pineapple cheese, homemade	5.6 oz	81	10	270
pumpkin, w/vegetable shortening crust	whole (9″ diam)	464	102	1,920
	⅙ pie	78	17	320
raisin, homemade	4.2 oz	22	13	325
rhubarb, homemade	5.6 oz	102	17	405
shoofly, homemade	3.9 oz	129	16	441

	Portion	Calcium (mg)	Total Fat (g)	Total Calor
strawberry, homemade	4 oz	18	9	228
sweet potato, homemade	5.6 oz	110	18	342

Pie Fillings *See* DESSERTS: CUSTARDS, GELATINS, PUDDINGS, & PIE FILLINGS

- **BRAND NAME**

Dromedary

date nut roll	½″ slice	20	2	80

Kellogg's
FROSTED POP-TARTS

blueberry	1	13	5	200
brown sugar cinnamon	1	?	7	210
chocolate fudge	1	?	4	200
Dutch apple	1	?	6	210
peanut butter & jelly	1	12	9	220

POP-TARTS

blueberry	1	14	5	210
brown sugar cinnamon	1	?	8	210

Nabisco

Frosted Toastettes or Toastettes, all flavors	1	<20	5	200

Pepperidge Farm Frozen Cakes & Pastries
FRUIT SQUARES

apple	1	<20	12	220
blueberry	1	<20	11	220
cherry	1	<20	12	230

LAYER CAKES

coconut	1⅝ oz	20	8	180
devil's food	1⅝ oz	20	8	170
German chocolate	1⅝ oz	20	10	180
golden	1⅝ oz	20	9	180
vanilla	1⅝ oz	20	8	170

OLD FASHIONED CAKES

butter pound	1 oz	20	6	120
carrot w/cream cheese icing	1⅜ oz	20	7	130

PUFF PASTRY

apple dumplings	3 oz	<20	13	260
apple strudel	3 oz	20	10	240
patty shells	1	<20	15	210
puff pastry sheets	¼ sheet	<20	17	260

	Portion	Calcium (mg)	Total Fat (g)	Total Calor
turnovers				
apple	1	<20	17	300
blueberry	1	<20	19	310
cherry	1	<20	19	310
peach	1	<20	18	310
raspberry	1	<20	17	310
SUPREME CAKES				
Boston cream	2⅞ oz	40	14	290
chocolate	2⅞ oz	40	16	300
Grand Marnier	1½ oz	20	18	160
lemon coconut	3 oz	20	13	280
raspberry mocha	3⅛ oz	20	14	310
strawberry cream	2 oz	20	7	190
Pillsbury				
sweet rolls, all flavors	1	0	?	210– 290
turnovers, all flavors	1	0	8	170
Rich's				
Bavarian cream puffs	1	9	8	146
chocolate éclairs	2 oz	10	10	205
Sara Lee				
ALL BUTTER COFFEE CAKES				
butter streusel	⅛ cake	12	7	160
cheese	⅛ cake	26	12	210
pecan	⅛ cake	14	8	160
ALL BUTTER POUND CAKES				
Original	¹⁄₁₀ cake	7	7	130
Family Size	¹⁄₁₅ cake	7	7	130
chocolate chip	¹⁄₁₀ cake	14	5	130
walnut raisin	¹⁄₁₀ cake	18	5	140
ELEGANT ENDINGS				
Classic	⅙ pkg	66	22	350
INDIVIDUAL DANISH				
apple	1	11	6	120
cheese	1	14	8	130
cinnamon raisin	1	17	8	150
raspberry	1	9	6	130
LE PASTRIE CROISSANTS				
apple	1	32	11	260
chocolate	1	48	18	320
cinnamon-nut-raisin	1	48	17	350
strawberry	1	33	11	270

	Portion	Calcium (mg)	Total Fat (g)	Total Calor
LIGHT CLASSICS				
French cheesecake				
plain	1/10 pkg	31	13	200
strawberry	1/10 pkg	29	11	200
mousse cake				
chocolate	1/10 pkg	27	14	200
strawberry	1/10 pkg	18	11	180
SINGLE-LAYER ICED CAKES				
banana	1/8 cake	7	6	170
carrot	1/8 cake	20	13	260
TWO-LAYER CAKES				
Black Forest	1/8 cake	21	8	190
strawberry shortcake	1/8 cake	23	8	190

❑ DESSERTS: CUSTARDS, GELATINS, PUDDINGS, & PIE FILLINGS

Custard

	Portion	Calcium (mg)	Total Fat (g)	Total Calor
plain				
baked, homemade	1/2 c	148	7	153
boiled, homemade	1/2 c	131	7	164
from mix	1/2 c	194	5	161
banana	1/2 c	142	5	143
chocolate	1/2 c	144	4	142
coconut	1/2 c	141	4	144
lemon	1/2 c	142	5	143
vanilla	1/2 c	142	5	143

Gelatin

	Portion	Calcium (mg)	Total Fat (g)	Total Calor
dry	1 envelope	1	tr	25
made w/water, all flavors	1/2 c	tr	tr	81
Bavarian (w/whipped cream)				
chocolate	1 serving	58	23	331
strawberry	1 serving	50	18	227

Pie Filling

	Portion	Calcium (mg)	Total Fat (g)	Total Calor
pumpkin pie mix, canned	1/2 c	49	tr	141

Pudding

	Portion	Calcium (mg)	Total Fat (g)	Total Calor
butterscotch, homemade	1/2 c	165	5	207

	Portion	Calcium (mg)	Total Fat (g)	Total Calor
chocolate				
canned	5 oz	74	11	205
from mix, prepared w/whole milk				
regular	½ c	146	4	150
instant	½ c	130	4	155
homemade	½ c	147	7	219
Indian, baked, homemade	⅔ c	221	6	161
lemon snow, homemade	½ c	4	tr	114
rice, from mix, prepared w/ whole milk	½ c	133	4	155
rice w/raisins, homemade	¾ c	142	5	212
tapioca				
canned	5 oz	119	5	160
from mix, prepared w/whole milk	½ c	131	4	145
homemade	½ c	105	5	133
vanilla				
canned	5 oz	79	10	220
from mix, prepared w/whole milk				
regular	½ c	132	4	145
instant	½ c	129	4	150
homemade	½ c	144	5	152

Rennin Dessert

	Portion	Calcium (mg)	Total Fat (g)	Total Calor
plain, homemade	½ c	141	4	113
chocolate, from mix				
prepared w/whole milk	½ c	159	18	127
prepared w/skim milk	½ c	163	1	95
fruit vanilla, from mix				
prepared w/whole milk	½ c	161	5	140
prepared w/skim milk	½ c	143	tr	88

• BRAND NAME

D-Zerta

	Portion	Calcium (mg)	Total Fat (g)	Total Calor
gelatin, low-cal	½ c	<20	0	8
pudding, reduced-calorie, prepared w/skim milk				
chocolate	½ c	150	0	60
vanilla	½ c	150	0	70

Jell-O
AMERICANA DESSERTS, PREPARED W/WHOLE MILK

	Portion	Calcium (mg)	Total Fat (g)	Total Calor
golden egg custard	½ c	200	5	160
rice pudding	½ c	150	4	170

	Portion	Calcium (mg)	Total Fat (g)	Total Calor
tapioca pudding				
chocolate	½ c	150	5	170
vanilla	½ c	150	4	160
GELATIN				
average values, all flavors	½ c	<20	0	80
PUDDING & PIE FILLING				
Regular, Prepared w/Whole Milk				
butterscotch	½ c	150	4	170
chocolate	½ c	150	4	160
vanilla	½ c	150	4	160
Instant, Prepared w/Whole Milk				
banana cream	½ c	150	4	160
butterscotch	½ c	150	4	160
chocolate	½ c	150	4	180
lemon	½ c	150	4	170
vanilla	½ c	150	4	170
Sugar-free, Prepared w/2% Low-Fat Milk				
chocolate	½ c	150	3	90
vanilla	½ c	150	2	80
Sugar-free Instant, Prepared w/2% Low-Fat Milk				
banana	½ c	150	2	90
butterscotch	½ c	150	2	90
chocolate	½ c	150	3	100
vanilla	½ c	150	2	90
RICH & DELICIOUS MOUSSE, PREPARED W/WHOLE MILK				
chocolate or chocolate fudge	½ c	100	6	150
Rich's Puddings				
butterscotch	3 oz	26	6	133
chocolate	3 oz	22	7	141
vanilla	3 oz	26	6	129
Royal				
GELATIN				
all flavors				
regular	½ c	<20	0	80
sugar-free	½ c	<20	0	6
PUDDING & PIE FILLING				
Cooked				
banana cream, prepared	½ c	150	4	160
butterscotch, prepared	½ c	150	4	160
chocolate				
dry	0.9 oz	<20	1	120
prepared	½ c	150	4	180

	Portion	Calcium (mg)	Total Fat (g)	Total Calor
custard, prepared	½ c	150	5	150
Dark 'n Sweet, prepared	½ c	150	4	180
flan w/caramel sauce, prepared	½ c	150	5	150
key lime, prepared	½ c	<20	3	160
lemon				
dry	½ oz	<20	0	50
prepared	½ c	<20	3	160
vanilla				
dry	0.7 oz	<20	1	80
prepared	½ c	150	4	160
Instant				
banana cream, prepared	½ c	150	5	180
butterscotch, prepared	½ c	150	5	180
chocolate				
dry	1 oz	<20	1	120
prepared	½ c	150	4	190
Dark 'n Sweet, prepared	½ c	150	4	190
lemon				
dry	0.8 oz	<20	1	110
prepared	½ c	150	5	180
pistachio nut, prepared	½ c	150	4	170
vanilla				
dry	0.8 oz	<20	1	100
prepared	½ c	150	5	180
Instant Sugar-free				
butterscotch, prepared	½ c	150	2	100
chocolate				
dry	½ oz	<20	0	50
prepared	½ c	150	3	110
vanilla				
dry	0.4 oz	<20	0	40
prepared	½ c	150	2	100

◻ DESSERTS, FROZEN: ICE CREAM, ICE MILK, ICES & SHERBETS, & FROZEN JUICE, PUDDING, TOFU, & YOGURT

Frozen Pudding on a Stick

banana	1	76	3	94
butterscotch	1	76	3	94
chocolate	1	86	3	99
chocolate fudge	1	88	3	99
vanilla	1	76	3	93

	Portion	Calcium (mg)	Total Fat (g)	Total Calor
Frozen Yogurt				
IN A CUP				
fruit varieties	½ c	100	1	108
ON A STICK				
raspberry, chocolate-coated	1	98	7	127
strawberry	1	78	1	69
Ice Cream				
chocolate	1 c	186	16	295
French custard	1 c	194	14	257
French vanilla, soft serve	1 c	236	23	377
strawberry	1 c	146	12	250
vanilla				
10% fat	1 c	176	14	269
16% fat	1 c	151	24	349
Ice Cream Novelties & Cones				
ice cream cone (cone only)	1	19	tr	45
ice cream sandwich	1	73	6	167
vanilla ice cream bar w/chocolate coating	1	70	11	162
vanilla ice milk bar w/chocolate coating	1	98	8	144
Ice Milk				
chocolate	⅔ c	140	5	137
strawberry	⅔ c	161	3	133
vanilla				
regular	1 c	176	6	184
soft serve	1 c	274	5	223
Ices & Sherbets				
lemon sherbet	¾ c	168	5	241
lime/orange ice	1 c	tr	tr	247
	⅔ c	tr	tr	165
orange sherbet	1 c	103	4	270
sherbet, various flavors	1 c	96	0	236
▪ **BRAND NAME**				
Baskin-Robbins Ice Cream & Sherbet				
chocolate	4 oz	115	13	264

	Portion	Calcium (mg)	Total Fat (g)	Total Calor
Chocolate Mousse Royale	4 oz	112	14	293
French vanilla	4 oz	127	19	290
orange sherbet	4 oz	35	2	158
Pralines 'n Cream	4 oz	99	13	283
raspberry sorbet	4 oz	0	0	134
Rocky Road	4 oz	94	11	291
strawberry	4 oz	101	10	226
vanilla	4 oz	136	13	235
wild strawberry (low-fat)	4 oz	175	2	90
Comet				
cups	1	<20	0	20
sugar cones	1	<20	0	40
Dole				
FRUIT & CREAM BARS				
blueberry	1	32	1	90
peach	1	27	1	90
strawberry	1	32	1	90
FRUIT 'N JUICE BARS				
banana	1	2	tr	80
orange w/mandarin	1	2	tr	70
piña colada	1	tr	3	90
pineapple	1	9	tr	70
raspberry	1	1	tr	70
strawberry	1	6	tr	70
SORBETS				
mandarin orange	4 oz	tr	tr	110
peach	4 oz	3	tr	120
pineapple	4 oz	9	tr	120
raspberry	4 oz	tr	tr	110
strawberry	4 oz	8	tr	110
Drumstick				
Drumstick sundae cone	1	67	10	186
Jell-O				
FRUIT BARS				
all flavors	1	<20	0	45
GELATIN POPS				
all flavors	1	<20	0	35
PUDDING POPS				
chocolate	1	60	2	80
chocolate-covered vanilla	1	60	7	130
vanilla w/chocolate chips	1	60	3	80

	Portion	Calcium (mg)	Total Fat (g)	Total Calor
Land O'Lakes				
ice cream, vanilla	4 fl oz	80	7	140
ice milk, vanilla	4 fl oz	80	3	90
sherbet, fruit flavors	4 fl oz	40	2	130
Life Savers				
Flavor Pops, all flavors	1	<20	0	40
Minute Maid Frozen Fruit Juice Bars				
cherry, fruit punch, grape, orange, strawberry (Variety Pack)	2¼ oz	<20	0 or tr	60
Snack Pack	1 oz	<20	0 or tr	25
Oreo Cookies 'n Cream				
ICE CREAM				
chocolate	3 fl oz	60	8	140
vanilla	3 fl oz	60	8	140
NOVELTIES				
on a stick	1	60	15	220
sandwich	1	80	11	240
Snackwich	1	<20	3	60
Popsicle				
Creamsicle	1	46	3	103
Fudgsicle	1	129	tr	91
Tofutti				
all flavors	4 oz	<20	<1– 14	90– 230

❑ DESSERT SAUCES, SYRUPS, & TOPPINGS

See also NUTS & NUT-BASED BUTTERS, FLOURS, MEALS, MILKS, PASTES, & POWDERS

Sauces, Syrups, & Flavored Toppings

	Portion	Calcium (mg)	Total Fat (g)	Total Calor
butterscotch sauce, homemade	2 T	41	7	203
butterscotch topping	3 T	24	tr	156
caramel topping	3 T	28	tr	155
cherry topping	3 T	14	tr	147
chocolate-flavored syrup or topping				
fudge type	2 T	38	5	125
thin type	2 T	6	tr	85
custard sauce, homemade	4 T	78	4	85
hard sauce, homemade	4 T	3	11	193

honey *See* SUGARS & SWEETENERS

	Portion	Calcium (mg)	Total Fat (g)	Total Calor
lemon sauce, homemade	4 T	3	3	133
pineapple topping	3 T	14	tr	146
walnuts in syrup topping	3 T	19	1	169

Whipped Cream & Whipped Cream–Type Toppings

nondairy				
powdered, prepared w/whole	1 T	4	1	8
milk	1 c	72	10	151
pressurized, containing	1 T	tr	1	11
lauric acid oil & sodium	1 c	4	16	184
caseinate				
semisolid, frozen, containing	1 T	tr	1	13
lauric acid oil & sodium	1 c	5	19	239
caseinate				
whipped cream topping, pres-	1 T	3	1	8
surized	1 c	61	13	154

▪ BRAND NAME

Cool Whip, Dream Whip, D-Zerta				
all	1 T	<20	0–1	8–16
Hershey				
chocolate fudge topping	2 T	20	4	100
Smucker's				
all	2 T	<20	?	100– 150

▢ DINNERS, FROZEN

▪ BRAND NAME

Hungry-Man Dinners *See* Swanson, *below*
Lean Cuisine *See* Stouffer, *below*
Le Menu

beef sirloin tips	11½ oz	80	19	410
beef Stroganoff	10 oz	80	26	450
breast of chicken parmigiana	11½ oz	150	19	390
chicken à la king	10¼ oz	60	13	330
chicken cordon bleu	11 oz	100	20	470
chicken Florentine	12½ oz	150	24	480
chopped sirloin beef	12¼ oz	20	19	410
ham steak	10 oz	60	11	310
pepper steak	11½ oz	40	14	380

	Portion	Calcium (mg)	Total Fat (g)	Total Calor
sliced breast of turkey w/ mushrooms	11¼ oz	40	23	460
stuffed flounder	10¼ oz	80	18	350
sweet & sour chicken	11¼ oz	80	23	460
vegetable lasagne	11 oz	200	19	360
Yankee pot roast	11 oz	40	15	360
Le Menu Light Style				
beef à l'orange	10 oz	60	8	290
chicken cacciatore	10 oz	80	8	260
flounder vin blanc	10 oz	80	5	220
glazed chicken breast	10 oz	60	5	240
3-cheese stuffed shells	10 oz	150	8	280
turkey divan	10 oz	100	9	280
L'Orient				
beef broccoli	11 oz	60	30	530
Cantonese chicken chow mein	11½ oz	60	5	280
Firecracker chicken	10½ oz	40	10	380
lemon chicken	11 oz	60	15	400
orange beef	10¾ oz	40	12	380
rock sugar–glazed pork	10¾ oz	60	15	360
Stouffer				
DINNER SUPREME				
baked chicken breast w/gravy	11 oz	40	9	330
beef teriyaki	11⅜ oz	40	13	370
beef tips Bourguignonne	12⅜ oz	100	15	360
chicken Florentine	11 oz	200	18	430
chicken w/Supreme Sauce	11⅜ oz	100	12	360
flounder w/dill cream sauce	11⅝ oz	80	19	370
flounder w/roasted red pepper sauce	12 oz	100	19	360
Salisbury steak w/gravy & mushrooms	13½ oz	150	18	380
LEAN CUISINE				
beef & pork cannelloni w/ Mornay sauce	9⅝ oz	200	10	270
breast of chicken Marsala w/ vegetables	8⅛ oz	20	5	190
cheese cannelloni w/tomato sauce	9⅛ oz	300	10	270
chicken à l'orange w/almond rice	8 oz	20	5	270
chicken & vegetables w/vermicelli	12¾ oz	100	7	270
chicken cacciatore w/vermicelli	10⅞ oz	40	10	280
chicken chow mein w/rice	11¼ oz	20	5	250
filet of fish divan	12⅜ oz	200	9	270
filet of fish Florentine	9 oz	150	9	240

	Portion	Calcium (mg)	Total Fat (g)	Total Calor
filet of fish jardiniere w/souffléed potatoes	11¼ oz	200	10	280
glazed chicken w/vegetable rice	8½ oz	20	8	270
herbed lamb w/rice	10⅜ oz	40	8	280
linguine w/clam sauce	9⅝ oz	20	7	260
meatball stew	10 oz	40	10	250
Oriental beef w/vegetables & rice	8⅝ oz	20	8	270
Oriental scallops & vegetables w/rice	11 oz	40	3	220
Salisbury steak w/Italian-style sauce & vegetables	9½ oz	150	13	270
shrimp & chicken Cantonese w/noodles	10⅛ oz	60	9	270
spaghetti w/beef & mushroom sauce	11½ oz	60	7	280
stuffed cabbage w/meat in tomato sauce	10¾ oz	80	9	220
tuna lasagna w/spinach noodles & vegetables	9¾ oz	250	10	280
turkey Dijon	9½ oz	100	10	280
veal lasagne	10¼ oz	250	8	280
veal primavera	9⅛ oz	60	9	250
zucchini lasagna	11 oz	300	7	260

Swanson
3-COMPARTMENT DINNERS

	Portion	Calcium (mg)	Total Fat (g)	Total Calor
beans & franks	10½ oz	55	17	420
macaroni & beef	12 oz	48	15	370
macaroni & cheese	12¼ oz	48	15	380
noodles & chicken	10½ oz	37	9	270
spaghetti & meatballs	12½ oz	100	15	370

4-COMPARTMENT DINNERS

	Portion	Calcium (mg)	Total Fat (g)	Total Calor
beans & franks	10½ oz	100	20	500
beef	11¼ oz	20	8	350
beef enchiladas	13¾ oz	80	24	480
beef in barbecue sauce	11 oz	80	15	460
chicken in barbecue sauce	11¾ oz	80	13	450
chicken nugget platter	8¾ oz	40	25	470
chopped sirloin beef	11 oz	80	20	380
fish & chips	10 oz	40	20	500
fish nugget	9½ oz	60	23	450
fried chicken				
barbecue-flavored	edible portion = 10 oz	100	27	580
dark meat	edible portion = 10 oz	60	28	580
white meat	edible portion = 10½ oz	100	27	580

	Portion	Calcium (mg)	Total Fat (g)	Total Calor
loin of pork	10¾ oz	40	12	310
meat loaf	10¾ oz	80	21	430
Mexican-style combination	14¼ oz	150	25	500
Polynesian style	12 oz	60	8	360
Salisbury steak	10¾ oz	60	18	410
sweet & sour chicken	12 oz	100	13	390
Swiss steak	10 oz	40	11	350
turkey	11½ oz	40	11	360
veal parmigiana	12¼ oz	150	23	460
Western style	11½ oz	60	21	440

HUNGRY-MAN DINNERS

	Portion	Calcium (mg)	Total Fat (g)	Total Calor
boneless chicken	17¾ oz	80	27	710
chicken nuggets	16 oz	40	26	600
chicken parmigiana	20 oz	300	51	810
chopped beef steak	16¾ oz	60	33	590
fish & chips	14¾ oz	100	39	780
fried chicken				
breast portions	14½ oz	60	50	930
dark portions	edible portion = 14½ oz	60	48	910
lasagna	18¾ oz	300	26	740
Mexican style	20¼ oz	300	39	750
Salisbury steak	18¼ oz	300	42	660
sliced beef	15½ oz	40	13	470
turkey	17 oz	80	18	550
veal parmigiana	18¼ oz	150	30	630
Western style	17½ oz	80	34	740

❑ EGGS & EGG SUBSTITUTES

Chicken Eggs

COOKED

egg dishes, prepared *See* BREAKFAST FOODS, PREPARED; FAST FOODS

	Portion	Calcium (mg)	Total Fat (g)	Total Calor
fried in butter	1 large	26	6	83
hard boiled	1 large	28	6	79
omelet, cooked w/butter & milk	1 egg (large)	47	7	95
poached	1 large	28	6	79
scrambled, w/butter & milk	1 large	47	7	95

DRIED

	Portion	Calcium (mg)	Total Fat (g)	Total Calor
whole	1 c sifted	180	36	505
whole, stabilized (glucose-reduced)	1 c sifted	189	37	523

	Portion	Calcium (mg)	Total Fat (g)	Total Calor
white only				
flakes, stabilized (glucose-reduced)	½ lb	189	tr	796
powder, stabilized (glucose-reduced)	1 c sifted	96	tr	402
yolk only	1 c sifted	189	41	460
UNCOOKED				
whole, fresh or frozen	1	28	6	79
white only, fresh or frozen	1	4	tr	16
yolk only, fresh	1	26	6	63
Eggs, Other				
duck	1	45	10	130
goose	1	?	19	267
quail	1	6	1	14
turkey	1	78	9	135
Egg Substitute				
frozen, containing egg white, corn oil, & nonfat dry milk	¼ c	44	7	96
liquid, containing egg white, soybean oil, & soy protein	1 c	133	8	211
powder, containing egg white solids, whole egg solids, sweet whey solids, nonfat dry milk, & soy protein	0.7 oz	65	3	88

- **BRAND NAME**

Fleischmann's				
Egg Beaters	¼ c	20	0	25
Egg Beaters w/Cheez	½ c	200	6	130

❑ ENTREES & MAIN COURSES, CANNED & BOXED

chili & bean products, canned & boxed *See* LEGUMES & LEGUME PRODUCTS; SOYBEANS & SOYBEAN PRODUCTS

	Portion	Calcium (mg)	Total Fat (g)	Total Calor

- **BRAND NAME**

Chun King
DIVIDER PAK ENTREES, CANNED

4 Servings/42 Oz Pkg

beef chow mein	7 oz	20	2	100
beef pepper Oriental	7 oz	20	4	110
chicken chow mein	7 oz	20	4	110
pork chow mein	7 oz	20	4	120
shrimp chow mein	7 oz	40	2	100

2 Servings/24 Oz Pkg

beef chow mein	8 oz	20	2	110
chicken chow mein	8 oz	20	4	120

STIR-FRY ENTREES, CANNED

chow mein w/beef	6 oz	20	19	290
chow mein w/chicken	6 oz	20	11	220
egg foo young	5 oz	40	8	140
pepper steak	6 oz	20	17	250
sukiyaki	6 oz	20	17	260

Franco-American

beef ravioli in meat sauce	7½ oz	20	5	230
macaroni & cheese	7⅜ oz	80	5	170
PizzO's	7½ oz	20	2	170
spaghetti in tomato sauce w/ cheese	7⅜ oz	20	2	190
SpaghettiO's in tomato & cheese sauce	7⅜ oz	20	2	170
spaghetti w/meatballs in to- mato sauce	7⅜ oz	20	8	220

Noodle-Roni Pasta

chicken & mushroom flavor, prepared	½ c	40	3	150
fettucini, prepared	½ c	40	17	300
garlic & butter, prepared	½ c	60	16	290
herbs & butter, prepared	½ c	20	7	160
parmesano, prepared	½ c	60	13	230
pesto Italiano, prepared	½ c	20	11	210
Rominoff, prepared	½ c	80	11	240
Stroganoff, prepared	¾ c	100	19	360

Swanson

chicken à la king	5¼ oz	40	12	180
chicken & dumplings	7½ oz	20	12	220
chicken stew	7⅝ oz	20	7	170

Van Camp's

Noodle Weenee	1 c	47	9	245
tamales w/sauce	1 c	36	16	293

	Portion	Calcium (mg)	Total Fat (g)	Total Calor

☐ ENTREES & MAIN COURSES, FROZEN

Celentano

	Portion	Calcium (mg)	Total Fat (g)	Total Calor
baked pasta & cheese	12 oz	700	21	530
broccoli stuffed shells	11½ oz	300	17	400
cannelloni Florentine	12 oz	300	17	380
cavatelli	3.2 oz	20	1	270
chicken cutlets parmigiana	9 oz	500	5	310
chicken primavera	11½ oz	20	9	270
eggplant parmigiana	8 oz	150	22	330
	7 oz	130	12	270
Eggplant Rollettes	11 oz	250	30	420
lasagne	8 oz	200	16	320
	6¼ oz	300	7	250
lasagne primavera	11 oz	250	9	300
manicotti				
w/sauce	8 oz	210	15	300
w/out sauce	7 oz	500	18	380
ravioli				
miniround cheese, w/out sauce	4 oz	80	6	250
round cheese, w/out sauce	6½ oz	230	12	410
stuffed shells				
w/sauce	8 oz	210	14	320
w/out sauce	6¼ oz	350	15	350

Lean Cuisine *See* Stouffer, *under* DINNERS, FROZEN

Le Menu Entrees

	Portion	Calcium (mg)	Total Fat (g)	Total Calor
beef burgundy	7½ oz	20	23	330
chicken Kiev	8 oz	40	39	530
manicotti	8½ oz	350	12	300
Oriental chicken	8½ oz	40	6	260

Mrs. Paul's

eggplant parmigiana *See* VEGETABLES, PLAIN & PREPARED

AU NATUREL SEAFOOD

	Portion	Calcium (mg)	Total Fat (g)	Total Calor
cod fillets	4 oz	<20	2	90
flounder fillets	4 oz	20	2	90
haddock fillets	4 oz	<20	1	80
perch fillets	4 oz	<20	2	80
sole fillets	4 oz	230	2	90

BUTTERED SEAFOOD

	Portion	Calcium (mg)	Total Fat (g)	Total Calor
fish fillets	2	20	9	170

LIGHT SEAFOOD ENTREES

	Portion	Calcium (mg)	Total Fat (g)	Total Calor
fish & pasta Florentine	9½ oz	250	9	240
fish au gratin	10 oz	300	8	290
fish Dijon	9½ oz	100	15	280

	Portion	Calcium (mg)	Total Fat (g)	Total Calor
fish Florentine	9 oz	300	4	210
fish Mornay	10 oz	100	14	280
shrimp & clams w/linguini	10 oz	20	6	280
shrimp Cajun style	10½ oz	40	4	200
shrimp Oriental	11 oz	80	5	280
shrimp primavera	11 oz	60	4	240
tuna pasta casserole	11 oz	350	7	290

PREPARED BATTERED SEAFOOD

	Portion	Calcium (mg)	Total Fat (g)	Total Calor
batter-dipped fish fillets	2	40	25	390
Crunchy Light Batter				
fish fillets	2	20	17	310
fish sticks	4	20	13	240
flounder fillets	2	20	16	310
haddock fillets	2	20	17	330
fried clams in a light batter	2½ oz	20	13	240

PREPARED BREADED SEAFOOD

	Portion	Calcium (mg)	Total Fat (g)	Total Calor
catfish fillets	1	<20	10	220
combination seafood platter	9 oz	80	31	590
Crispy Crunchy				
fish fillets	2	40	16	280
fish sticks	4	<20	10	200
flounder fillets	2	20	15	270
haddock fillets	2	20	12	250
perch fillets	2	20	19	320
deviled crabs	1 piece	80	8	190
fish cakes	2	60	11	250
french-fried scallops	3½ oz	40	9	230
fried shrimp	3 oz	40	11	200
Supreme Light Breaded				
fish fillets	1	20	13	290
flounder or sole fillets	1	40	13	280

Sara Lee Le Sandwich Croissants

	Portion	Calcium (mg)	Total Fat (g)	Total Calor
cheddar cheese	1	251	23	380
chicken & broccoli	1	106	17	340
ham & Swiss cheese	1	154	18	340
turkey, bacon, & cheese	1	156	20	370

Stouffer
ENTREES

	Portion	Calcium (mg)	Total Fat (g)	Total Calor
beef & spinach stuffed pasta shells w/tomato sauce	9 oz	150	12	300
beef chop suey w/rice	12 oz	20	12	340
beef pie	10 oz	40	37	560
beef stew	10 oz	20	16	310
beef Stroganoff w/parsley noodles	9¾ oz	60	21	410
beef teriyaki in sauce w/rice & vegetables	9¾ oz	40	9	330

	Portion	Calcium (mg)	Total Fat (g)	Total Calor
cashew chicken in sauce w/ rice	9½ oz	20	17	410
cheese soufflé	7⅝ oz	400	36	480
cheese stuffed pasta shells w/ meat sauce	9 oz	400	16	340
chicken à la king w/rice	9½ oz	80	11	320
chicken chow mein w/out noodles	8 oz	20	5	140
chicken crêpes w/mushroom sauce	8¼ oz	150	21	370
chicken divan	8½ oz	200	22	350
chicken paprikash w/egg noo- dles	10½ oz	60	15	390
chicken pie	10 oz	80	34	530
chicken stuffed pasta shells w/cheese sauce	9 oz	350	24	420
chili con carne w/beans	8¾ oz	80	11	280
creamed chicken	6½ oz	60	24	320
creamed chipped beef	5½ oz	100	17	240
escalloped chicken & noo- dles	5¾ oz	40	16	260
fettucini Alfredo	5 oz	150	20	280
fettucini primavera	½ of 10⅝ oz pkg	150	21	270
green pepper steak w/rice	10½ oz	20	11	340
Ham & Asparagus Bake	9½ oz	200	35	510
ham & asparagus crêpes	6¼ oz	150	18	310
ham & Swiss cheese crêpes w/cream sauce	7½ oz	400	26	410
lasagna	10½ oz	250	13	370
linguini w/pesto sauce	½ of 8¼ oz pkg	150	10	210
lobster Newburg	6½ oz	100	30	360
macaroni & beef w/tomatoes	11½ oz	60	16	360
macaroni & cheese	6 oz	200	12	250
noodles Romanoff	4 oz	60	9	170
roast beef hash	5¾ oz	<20	15	250
Salisbury steaks w/onion gravy	6 oz	20	14	230
Scallops & Shrimp Mariner w/ Rice	10¼ oz	150	18	390
short ribs of beef w/vegetable gravy	5¾ oz	<20	20	280
spaghetti w/meatballs	12⅝ oz	150	13	370
spaghetti w/meat sauce	14 oz	100	15	440
spinach crêpes w/cheddar cheese sauce	9½ oz	300	27	420
steak & mushroom pie	10 oz	20	24	430
stuffed green peppers w/beef in tomato sauce	7¾ oz	150	11	220

	Portion	Calcium (mg)	Total Fat (g)	Total Calor
Swedish meatballs in gravy w/parsley noodles	11 oz	60	25	470
tuna noodle casserole	5¾ oz	80	8	190
turkey casserole w/gravy & dressing	9¾ oz	100	19	380
turkey pie	10 oz	80	35	540
turkey tetrazzini	6 oz	60	14	230
vegetable lasagna	10½ oz	500	25	450
Welsh rarebit	5 oz	400	30	360

LEAN CUISINE See Stouffer, *under* DINNERS, FROZEN

Swanson
CHICKEN DUET ENTREES

	Portion	Calcium (mg)	Total Fat (g)	Total Calor
creamy broccoli	6 oz	40	17	310
creamy green bean	6 oz	60	18	330
saucy tomato	6 oz	150	18	340
savory wild rice	6 oz	40	14	290

CHICKEN DUET GOURMET NUGGETS

	Portion	Calcium (mg)	Total Fat (g)	Total Calor
ham & cheese	3 oz	100	13	220
Mexican style	3 oz	80	13	220
pizza style	3 oz	60	12	210
spinach & herb	3 oz	80	13	230

CHUNKY PIES

	Portion	Calcium (mg)	Total Fat (g)	Total Calor
beef	10 oz	20	29	550
chicken	10 oz	40	33	580
turkey	10 oz	20	31	540

DIPSTERS

	Portion	Calcium (mg)	Total Fat (g)	Total Calor
barbecue	3 oz	<20	13	220
Coconola	3 oz	<20	15	240
herb	3 oz	<20	14	220
Italian style	3 oz	40	16	230

ENTREES

	Portion	Calcium (mg)	Total Fat (g)	Total Calor
Chicken Nibbles	edible portion = 5 oz	<20	18	260
Fish 'n' Fries	7¼ oz	40	21	420
fried chicken	edible portion = 6½ oz	20	19	300
Salisbury steak	10 oz	200	32	410
Swedish meatballs	9¼ oz	100	30	420
turkey	8¾ oz	40	11	270
veal parmigiana	10 oz	100	15	280

HUNGRY-MAN POT PIES

	Portion	Calcium (mg)	Total Fat (g)	Total Calor
beef	16 oz	60	33	680
chicken	16 oz	80	41	730

	Portion	Calcium (mg)	Total Fat (g)	Total Calor
turkey	16 oz	80	38	690
MAIN COURSE ENTREES				
lasagna w/meat	13¼ oz	250	19	470
macaroni & cheese	12 oz	250	16	390
PLUMP & JUICY				
chicken cutlets	3 oz	<20	12	200
Chicken Dipsters	3 oz	<20	14	220
Chicken Drumlets	3 oz	<20	14	220
Chicken Nibbles	3¼ oz	20	20	300
Extra Crispy fried chicken	3 oz	20	16	250
fried chicken				
assorted pieces	3¼ oz	20	17	270
breast portions	4½ oz	20	21	360
Take-Out fried chicken, assorted pieces	3¼ oz	20	17	270
thighs & drumsticks	3¼ oz	20	19	280
POT PIES				
beef	8 oz	40	21	410
chicken	8 oz	40	26	420
macaroni & cheese	7 oz	150	9	220
turkey	8 oz	20	24	410
Tyson				
chicken cordon bleu	about 3½ oz	96	13	225
chicken Kiev	about 3½ oz	9	22	290
stuffed chicken breast	about 3½ oz	23	7	160

◻ FAST FOODS

shakes				
chocolate	10 fl oz	319	11	360
strawberry	10 fl oz	320	8	319
vanilla	10 fl oz	344	8	314
tacos	1	109	11	195

▪ BRAND NAME

Arby's
DESSERTS

apple turnover	1	<20	18	303
cherry turnover	1	<20	18	280

	Portion	Calcium (mg)	Total Fat (g)	Total Calor
SANDWICHES				
Bac'n Cheddar Deluxe	1	150	37	526
Beef'n Cheddar	1	60	27	455
chicken breast	1	80	29	509
chicken club	1	?	32	621
chicken salad	1	?	20	386
fish fillet	1	40	32	580
hot ham & cheese	1	200	14	292
Philly Beef 'n Swiss	1	450	28	460
roast beef				
junior	1	40	9	218
regular	1	80	15	353
king	1	100	19	467
giant	1	100	23	531
super	1	100	22	501
Turkey Deluxe	1	80	17	375
SHAKES				
chocolate	1	250	12	451
Jamocha	1	250	11	368
vanilla	1	300	12	330
SIDE DISHES				
french fries	1 serving	<20	10	215
potato cakes	1 serving	<20	13	201
rice pilaf	1 serving	?	2	123
Scandinavian vegetables in sauce	1 serving	?	2	56
Burger King				
BREAKFAST ITEMS				
Breakfast Croissan'wich	1	?	19	304
w/bacon	1	136	24	355
w/ham	1	136	20	335
w/sausage	1	145	41	538
French toast sticks	1 serving	77	29	499
Great Danish	1	91	36	500
scrambled egg platter	1	101	30	468
w/bacon	1	103	36	536
w/sausage	1	112	52	702
BURGERS & SANDWICHES				
bacon double cheeseburger	1	168	31	510
cheeseburger	1	102	15	317
Chicken Specialty	1	79	40	688
Ham & Cheese Specialty	1	195	23	471
hamburger	1	37	12	275
Whaler fish	1	46	27	488
Whopper	1	84	36	628
w/cheese	1	215	43	711

	Portion	Calcium (mg)	Total Fat (g)	Total Calor
Whopper Jr.	1	40	17	322
w/cheese	1	105	20	364

CHICKEN

	Portion	Calcium (mg)	Total Fat (g)	Total Calor
Chicken Tenders	6 pieces	18	10	204

DESSERTS

	Portion	Calcium (mg)	Total Fat (g)	Total Calor
apple pie	1 slice	<20	12	305

SALADS

	Portion	Calcium (mg)	Total Fat (g)	Total Calor
plain salad	1 serving	37	0	28
w/bleu cheese dressing	1 serving	66	16	184
w/house dressing	1 serving	42	13	158
w/reduced-calorie Italian dressing	1 serving	40	0	42
w/Thousand Island dressing	1 serving	44	12	145

SHAKES

	Portion	Calcium (mg)	Total Fat (g)	Total Calor
chocolate	1 regular	260	12	320
syrup added	1 regular	248	11	374
vanilla	1 regular	295	10	321
syrup added	1 regular	?	10	334

SIDE DISHES

	Portion	Calcium (mg)	Total Fat (g)	Total Calor
french fries	1 regular serving	<20	13	227
onion rings	1 regular serving	124	16	274

Hardee's
BREAKFAST ITEMS

	Portion	Calcium (mg)	Total Fat (g)	Total Calor
American cheese slice	1	71	3	47
bacon & egg biscuit	1	206	26	410
Big Country Breakfast bacon	1 serving	150	50	761
Big Country Breakfast ham	1 serving	202	38	665
Big Country Breakfast sausage	1 serving	198	70	849
biscuit gravy	1 serving	19	10	144
Canadian Sunrise biscuit	1	286	30	482
cinnamon & raisin biscuit	1	103	16	276
cheese biscuit	1	155	16	304
country ham biscuit	1	169	18	323
egg	1	19	6	79
egg biscuit	1	184	19	336
ham biscuit	1	167	14	300
Hash Rounds potatoes	1 serving	9	16	249
jam	1 serving	4	0	51
Rise 'n' Shine biscuit	1	163	12	257
sausage & egg biscuit	1	196	35	503
sausage biscuit	1	190	28	426
steak biscuit	1	192	28	491

	Portion	Calcium (mg)	Total Fat (g)	Total Calor
BURGERS & SANDWICHES				
bacon cheeseburger	1	78	33	556
big deluxe burger	1	100	29	503
cheeseburger				
regular	1	95	15	327
¼ lb	1	94	28	511
chicken fillet	1	39	17	446
Fisherman's Fillet	1	139	20	469
hamburger	1	25	9	244
hot dog	1	33	14	285
hot ham & cheese	1	166	10	316
mushroom & Swiss burger	1	111	23	509
roast beef				
regular	1	10	12	312
big	1	15	22	440
turkey club	1	39	22	426
DESSERTS				
apple turnover	1	0	13	87
Big Cookie Treat	1	16	15	54
Cool Twist cone	1	?	5	164
SALADS				
chef salad	1	244	13	309
garden salad, w/Thousand Island dressing	1	?	34	501
side salad	1	14	tr	90
SHAKES				
chocolate	1	450	10	390
SIDE DISHES				
french fries	1 regular serving	9	12	252
	1 large serving	14	23	438
Jack-In-the-Box				
BEVERAGES				
hot chocolate	1	20	4	133
BREAKFAST ITEMS				
Breakfast Jack	1	170	13	307
grape jelly	1 serving	170	0	38
pancake platter	1	100	22	612
pancake syrup	1 serving	<20	0	121
scrambled egg platter	1	200	40	662

	Portion	Calcium (mg)	Total Fat (g)	Total Calor
BURGERS & SANDWICHES				
bacon cheeseburger	1	280	39	705
cheeseburger	1	60	17	325
Chicken Supreme	1	100	36	575
club pita, w/out sauce	1	40	8	277
ham & Swiss burger	1	280	49	754
hamburger	1	40	13	288
Hot Club Supreme	1	200	28	524
Jumbo Jack	1	140	34	584
w/cheese	1	270	40	677
Moby Jack	1	160	25	444
Monterey burger	1	270	57	808
mushroom burger	1	250	24	513
Swiss & bacon burger	1	220	47	678
Ultimate Cheeseburger	1	600	69	942
CRESCENT ROLLS				
Canadian crescent	1	130	31	452
sausage crescent	1	170	43	584
Supreme crescent	1	150	40	547
DESSERTS				
cheesecake	1 piece	110	18	309
hot apple turnover	1	<20	24	410
ENTREES				
chicken strip dinner	1	80	29	674
shrimp dinner	1	300	33	677
sirloin steak dinner	1	200	27	702
MEXICAN DISHES				
Fajita Pita	1	300	7	278
guacamole	1 serving	20	5	55
nachos				
cheese	1 serving	370	35	571
Supreme	1 serving	700	45	787
salsa	1 serving	<20	<1	8
taco	1	100	11	191
Super taco	1	150	17	288
PIZZA				
Pizza Pocket	1	100	28	497
SALAD DRESSINGS				
bleu cheese	1 serving	<20	11	131
buttermilk house	1 serving	<20	18	181
reduced-calorie French	1 serving	<20	4	80
Thousand Island	1 serving	<20	15	156

	Portion	Calcium (mg)	Total Fat (g)	Total Calor
SALADS				
chef salad	1	150	18	295
pasta & seafood salad	1	210	22	394
side salad	1	60	3	51
taco salad	1	280	24	377
SAUCES				
A-1 Steak	1 serving	<20	<1	18
BBQ	1 serving	<20	<1	39
Mayo-Mustard	1 serving	<20	13	124
Mayo-Onion	1 serving	<20	15	143
Seafood Cocktail	1 serving	<20	<1	57
SHAKES				
chocolate	1	350	7	330
strawberry	1	350	7	320
vanilla	1	350	6	320
SIDE DISHES				
french fries	1 regular serving	<20	12	221
	1 large serving	<20	19	353
onion rings	1 serving	30	23	382
Kentucky Fried Chicken				
FRIED CHICKEN				
Original Recipe				
breast				
center	1	39	14	257
side	1	48	17	276
drumstick	1	13	9	147
thigh	1	28	19	278
wing	1	38	12	181
Extra Crispy				
breast				
center	1	35	21	353
side	1	32	24	354
drumstick	1	15	11	173
thigh	1	46	26	371
wing	1	21	16	218
NUGGETS & SAUCES				
nuggets	1	2	3	46
barbecue sauce	1 oz	6	1	35
honey sauce	½ oz	1	<1	49
mustard sauce	1 oz	10	1	36
sweet & sour sauce	1 oz	5	1	58

	Portion	Calcium (mg)	Total Fat (g)	Total Calor
SIDE DISHES				
baked beans	1 serving	54	1	105
buttermilk biscuits	1	77	14	269
chicken gravy	1 serving	9	4	59
cole slaw	1 serving	29	6	103
corn on the cob	1 ear	7	3	176
Kentucky fries	1 serving	24	13	268
mashed potatoes	1 serving	21	1	59
w/gravy	1 serving	19	1	62
potato salad	1 serving	10	9	141
McDonald's				
BREAKFAST ITEMS				
biscuit				
w/bacon, cheese, & egg	1	2	32	483
w/biscuit spread	1	74	18	330
w/sausage	1	82	31	467
w/sausage & egg	1	119	40	585
danish				
apple	1	14	18	389
cinnamon raisin	1	35	21	445
iced cheese	1	33	22	395
raspberry	1	14	16	414
Egg McMuffin	1	226	16	340
English muffin w/butter	1	117	5	186
hash brown potatoes	1 serving	5	9	144
hotcakes w/butter syrup	1 serving	103	10	500
pork sausage	1 serving	16	19	210
Sausage McMuffin	1	168	26	427
w/egg	1	196	33	517
BURGERS & SANDWICHES				
Big Mac	1	203	35	570
cheeseburger	1	169	16	318
Filet-o-Fish	1	133	26	435
hamburger	1	84	11	263
McD.L.T.	1	250	44	680
Quarter Pounder	1	98	24	427
w/cheese	1	255	32	525
CHICKEN NUGGETS & SAUCES				
Chicken McNuggets	2	11	20	323
barbecue sauce	1 serving	4	tr	60
honey	1 serving	1	tr	50
hot mustard sauce	1 serving	8	2	63
sweet & sour sauce	1 serving	2	tr	64

	Portion	Calcium (mg)	Total Fat (g)	Total Calor
DESSERTS				
apple pie	1 piece	14	14	253
cookies				
Chocolaty Chip	1 serving	29	16	342
McDonaldland	1 serving	12	11	308
soft-serve ice cream & cone	1 serving	183	5	189
sundaes				
hot caramel	1	200	10	361
hot fudge	1	215	11	357
strawberry	1	174	9	320
SALAD BAR ITEMS				
bacon bits	1 serving	1	1	15
chef salad	1	222	13	226
chicken salad Oriental	1	47	4	146
chow mein noodles	1 serving	2	2	45
croutons	1 serving	6	2	52
garden salad	1	104	6	91
shrimp salad	1	64	3	99
side salad	1	47	3	48
SALAD DRESSINGS				
bleu cheese	½ pkg	37	17	171
French	½ pkg	2	10	114
house	½ pkg	10	17	163
lite vinaigrette	½ pkg	8	1	25
Oriental	½ pkg	7	2	51
Thousand Island	½ pkg	7	20	198
SHAKES				
chocolate	1	320	9	383
strawberry	1	322	9	362
vanilla	1	329	8	352
SIDE DISHES				
french fries	1 regular serving	9	12	220
Roy Rogers *BEVERAGES*				
hot chocolate	1	80	2	123
BREAKFAST ITEMS				
crescent roll	1	52	18	287
crescent sandwich	1	161	27	401
w/bacon	1	164	30	431
w/ham	1	167	42	557
w/sausage	1	163	29	449
egg & biscuit platter	1	117	27	394

	Portion	Calcium (mg)	Total Fat (g)	Total Calor
w/bacon	1	120	30	435
w/ham	1	120	29	442
w/sausage	1	123	41	550
pancake platter, w/syrup & butter	1	91	15	452
w/bacon	1	94	18	493
w/ham	1	94	17	506
w/sausage	1	97	30	608

BURGERS & SANDWICHES

	Portion	Calcium (mg)	Total Fat (g)	Total Calor
bacon cheeseburger	1	343	39	581
cheeseburger	1	340	37	563
hamburger	1	90	28	456
roast beef				
regular	1	87	10	317
w/cheese	1	337	19	424
large	1	89	12	360
w/cheese	1	339	21	467
RR Bar Burger	1	343	39	611

CHICKEN

	Portion	Calcium (mg)	Total Fat (g)	Total Calor
breast	1	23	24	412
breast & wing	1 each	31	37	604
drumstick/leg	1	6	8	140
nuggets	6	?	17	267
thigh	1	14	20	296
thigh & leg	1 each	20	28	436
wing	1	8	13	192

DESSERTS

	Portion	Calcium (mg)	Total Fat (g)	Total Calor
brownie	1	25	11	264
danish				
apple	1	100	12	249
cheese	1	37	12	254
cherry	1	39	14	271
strawberry shortcake	1 serving	274	19	447
sundaes				
caramel	1	204	9	293
hot fudge	1	264	13	337
strawberry	1	210	7	216

SALAD BAR ITEMS & SALAD DRESSINGS
Calcium values are not available.

SHAKES

	Portion	Calcium (mg)	Total Fat (g)	Total Calor
chocolate	1	290	10	358
strawberry	1	284	10	315
vanilla	1	300	11	306

	Portion	Calcium (mg)	Total Fat (g)	Total Calor
SIDE DISHES				
biscuit	1	64	12	231
cole slaw	1 serving	34	7	110
french fries	1 regular serving	18	14	268
	1 large serving	25	18	357
hot topped potato				
plain	1	20	tr	211
w/bacon & cheese	1	150	22	397
w/broccoli & cheese	1	210	18	376
w/oleo	1	23	7	274
w/sour cream & chives	1	96	21	408
w/taco beef & cheese	1	150	22	463
macaroni	1 serving	10	11	186
potato salad	1 serving	13	6	107
Wendy's				
BEVERAGES				
hot chocolate	1	60	1	110
lemonade	1	<20	<1	160
BREAKFAST ITEMS				
bacon	1 strip	<20	2	30
breakfast sandwich	1	150	19	370
buttermilk biscuit	1	100	17	320
danish				
apple	1	60	14	360
cheese	1	80	21	430
cinnamon raisin	1	60	18	410
French toast	2 slices	80	19	400
French toast toppings				
apple	1 pkt	<20	<1	130
blueberry	1 pkt	<20	<1	60
fried egg	1	20	6	90
grape jelly	1 pkt	<20	<1	40
omelet #1: ham & cheese	1	100	21	290
omelet #2: ham, cheese, & mushroom	1	100	17	250
omelet #3: ham, cheese, onion, & green pepper	1	150	19	280
omelet #4: mushroom, green pepper, & onion	1	60	15	210
potatoes	1 serving	20	22	360
sausage gravy	6 oz	40	36	440
sausage patty	1	<20	18	200
scrambled eggs	2 eggs	60	12	190
strawberry jam	1 pkt	<20	<1	40
syrup	1 pkt	<20	<1	140

	Portion	Calcium (mg)	Total Fat (g)	Total Calor
toast, w/margarine				
wheat	2 slices	<20	8	190
white	2 slices	20	9	250

BURGER & SANDWICH COMPONENTS

	Portion	Calcium (mg)	Total Fat (g)	Total Calor
American cheese slice	1	150	6	60
bacon	1 strip	<20	2	30
buns				
kaiser	1	20	2	180
multigrain	1	<20	3	140
white	1	40	2	140
catsup	1 t	<20	<1	6
hamburger patty, ¼ lb	1	<20	14	210
lettuce	1 leaf	<20	<1	2
mayonnaise	1 T	<20	10	90
mustard	1 t	<20	<1	4
onion	3 rings	<20	<1	2
pickles, dill	4 slices	<20	<1	2
taco sauce	1 pkt	<20	<1	10
tartar sauce	1 T	<20	9	80
tomatoes	1 slice	<20	<1	2

BURGERS & SANDWICHES

	Portion	Calcium (mg)	Total Fat (g)	Total Calor
Big Classic (two ¼-lb hamburger patties, mayonnaise, catsup, pickles, onion, tomatoes, lettuce, kaiser bun)	1	40	25	470
chicken breast fillet	1	<20	10	200
chicken fried steak	1	60	41	580
fish fillet	1	<20	11	210
Kids' Meal hamburger	1	40	9	200

CHICKEN NUGGETS & SAUCES

	Portion	Calcium (mg)	Total Fat (g)	Total Calor
Crispy Nuggets				
cooked in animal/vegetable oil	6	20	21	290
cooked in vegetable oil	6	20	21	310
barbecue sauce	1 pkt	<20	<1	50
honey	1 pkt	<20	<1	45
sweet & sour sauce	1 pkt	<20	<1	45
sweet mustard sauce	1 pkt	<20	1	50

CHILI

	Portion	Calcium (mg)	Total Fat (g)	Total Calor
chili	1 regular serving	60	8	240

	Portion	Calcium (mg)	Total Fat (g)	Total Calor
CONDIMENTS, SAUCES, & MISCELLANEOUS ITEMS				
catsup, half & half, hot chili seasoning, nondairy creamer, sugar	1 serving	<20	≤1	varies
cheese sauce	2 oz	150	12	140
margarine				
liquid	½ oz	?	11	100
whipped	1 T	?	8	70
sour cream	2 t	<20	2	20
DESSERTS				
chocolate chip cookie	1	<20	17	320
Frosty dairy dessert	1 regular serving	300	14	400
SALAD BAR ITEMS				
alfalfa sprouts	1 oz	<20	<1	8
American cheese	1 oz	200	7	90
bacon bits	⅛ oz	<20	<1	10
blueberries	1 T	<20	<1	6
bread sticks	2	<20	1	35
broccoli	½ c	60	<1	12
cabbage, red	¼ c	<20	<1	4
cantaloupe	2 pieces	<20	<1	18
carrots	¼ c	<20	<1	10
cauliflower	½ c	<20	<1	12
celery	1 T	<20	<1	0
cheddar cheese	1 oz	20	6	80
cherry peppers	1 T	<20	<1	6
chow mein noodles	½ oz	<20	4	70
cole slaw	¼ c	20	5	80
cottage cheese	½ c	60	4	110
croutons	½ oz	<20	3	60
cucumbers	4 slices	<20	<1	2
eggs	1 T	<20	2	30
grapefruit	2 oz	<20	<1	10
grapes	¼ c	<20	<1	30
green peas	1 oz	<20	<1	25
green peppers	¼ c	<20	<1	8
honeydew melon	2 pieces	<20	<1	20
jalapeño peppers	1 T	<20	<1	9
lettuce				
iceberg	1 c	<20	<1	8
romaine	1 c	40	<1	10
mozzarella cheese	1 oz	200	7	90
mushrooms	¼ c	<20	<1	4
oranges	2 oz	20	<1	25
Parmesan cheese, grated	1 oz	400	9	130
pasta salad	¼ c	<20	6	130
peaches	2 slices	<20	<1	17

	Portion	Calcium (mg)	Total Fat (g)	Total Calor
pepper rings	1 T	20	<1	2
pineapple chunks	½ c	<20	<1	70
provolone cheese	1 oz	200	7	90
radishes	½ oz	<20	<1	2
red onions	3 rings	<20	<1	2
strawberries	2 oz	<20	<1	18
sunflower seeds & raisins	1 oz	20	10	140
Swiss cheese	1 oz	200	7	90
tomatoes	1 oz	<20	<1	6
turkey ham	¼ c	?	2	50
watermelon	2 pieces	<20	<1	18

SALAD DRESSINGS

all regular	1 T	<20	4–7	50–70
all reduced-calorie	1 T	<20	2–5	25–50

SIDE DISHES

french fries				
cooked in animal/vegetable oil	1 regular serving	<20	15	310
cooked in vegetable oil	1 regular serving	<20	15	300
hot stuffed baked potatoes				
plain	1	40	2	250
bacon & cheese	1	200	30	570
broccoli & cheese	1	250	25	500
cheese	1	350	34	590
chili & cheese	1	250	20	510
sour cream & chives	1	40	24	460

TACO SALAD

taco salad	1 serving	300	19	430
taco sauce	1 pkt	<20	<1	10

❑ FATS, OILS, & SHORTENINGS
See also BUTTER & MARGARINE SPREADS

animal fats, all	1 T	?	13	115–116
shortening	1 T	?	13–14	113–120
vegetable oils, all	1 T	?	14	120

▪ BRAND NAME

Mazola

corn oil	1 T	<20	14	120
No-Stick	2½-second spray	<20	1	6

	Portion	Calcium (mg)	Total Fat (g)	Total Calor
Planters				
peanut oil	1 T	?	14	120

❏ FISH *See* SEAFOOD & SEAFOOD PRODUCTS

❏ FLOURS & CORNMEALS
See also NUTS & NUT-BASED BUTTERS, FLOURS, MEALS, MILKS, PASTES, & POWDERS; SEEDS & SEED-BASED BUTTERS, FLOURS, & MEALS

	Portion	Calcium (mg)	Total Fat (g)	Total Calor
arrowroot flour	1 T	0	0	29
buckwheat flour				
dark	1 oz	9	1	92
light, sifted	1 c	11	1	340
carob flour	1 T	28	tr	14
	1 c	359	1	185
corn flour, sifted	1 c	7	3	405
masa harina	⅓ c	77	2	137
masa trigo	⅓ c	66	4	149
white, tortilla, lime-treated	1 oz	25	2	103
yellow, tortilla, untreated	1 oz	4	1	101
corn germ, toasted	1 oz	3	7	130
cornmeal				
whole-ground, dry				
bolted	1 c	21	4	122
unbolted	1 c	24	5	122
degermed, enriched				
dry	1 c	8	2	138
cooked	1 c	2	tr	240
white, self-rising, dry	1 oz or ⅙ c	109	1	98
manioc (cassava) flour	3½ oz	148	1	320
potato flour	1 c	59	1	628
rice bran	1 oz	16	tr	80
rice flour	1 c	11	tr	479
rice polish	1 oz	17	2	101
rye flour				
dark	3½ oz	54	3	327
light	3½ oz	22	1	357
soy flour *See* SOYBEANS & SOYBEAN PRODUCTS				
wheat & gluten flour	1 c	56	3	529
wheat flour, enriched				
all-purpose				
sifted	1 c	18	1	420

	Portion	Calcium (mg)	Total Fat (g)	Total Calor
unsifted	1 c	20	1	455
bread, sifted	1 c	18	1	409
cake or pastry, sifted	1 c	16	1	350
self-rising, unsifted	1 c	331	1	440
whole-wheat & soy flour	3½ oz	684	7	365
whole-wheat flour, from hard wheats	1 c	49	2	400
whole-wheat flour, straight, soft	3½ oz	20	1	364

▪ BRAND NAME

Argo
	Portion	Calcium (mg)	Total Fat (g)	Total Calor
Argo & Kingsford's corn starch	1 T	<20	0	30

Arrowhead Mills
	Portion	Calcium (mg)	Total Fat (g)	Total Calor
barley flour	2 oz	20	1	200
brown rice flour	2 oz	20	1	200
buckwheat flour	2 oz	20	1	190
corn flour, yellow	2 oz	?	2	210
cornmeal				
blue	2 oz	<20	3	210
hi-lysine	2 oz	<20	2	210
yellow	2 oz	<20	2	210
Ezekiel flour	2 oz	20	1	200
millet flour	2 oz	20	2	185
oat flour	2 oz	20	1	200
pastry flour	2 oz	20	1	180
rye flour	2 oz	40	1	190
triticale flour	2 oz	20	1	190
unbleached white flour	2 oz	<20	1	200
vital wheat gluten	1 oz	<20	1	100
whole-wheat flour	2 oz	20	1	200

Aunt Jemima
CORNMEAL
	Portion	Calcium (mg)	Total Fat (g)	Total Calor
bolted white, mix	⅙ c	60	1	99
bolted yellow, mix	⅙ c	60	tr	97
buttermilk self-rising white, mix	3 T	60	1	101
enriched white	3 T	1	1	102
enriched yellow	3 T	1	1	102
self-rising white	⅙ c	109	1	98
self-rising white enriched bolted	⅙ c	109	1	99

	Portion	Calcium (mg)	Total Fat (g)	Total Calor
FLOUR				
enriched self-rising	¼ c	60	tr	109
Fearn				
rice flour	½ c	20	0	270
Heckers				
flour	about 1 c or 4 oz	200	1	380–400
Quaker Oats				
masa harina de maiz	⅓ c	77	2	137
masa trigo	⅓ c	66	4	149

❑ **FRANKFURTERS** *See* PROCESSED MEAT & POULTRY PRODUCTS

❑ **FRUIT, FRESH & PROCESSED**
See also PICKLES, OLIVES, RELISHES, & CHUTNEYS; SNACKS

	Portion	Calcium (mg)	Total Fat (g)	Total Calor
acerolas, raw	1 c	12	tr	31
apples				
raw				
w/skin	1 fruit = 4.9 oz	10	tr	81
w/out skin	1 fruit = 4½ oz	5	tr	72
baked in microwave, w/out skin	½ c sliced	4	tr	48
boiled, w/out skin	½ c sliced	4	tr	46
canned, sweetened, un-heated	½ c sliced	4	1	68
dehydrated, sulfured				
cooked	½ c	4	tr	71
uncooked	½ c	6	tr	104
dried, sulfured				
cooked, w/added sugar	½ c	4	tr	116
cooked, w/out added sugar	½ c	4	tr	72
uncooked	2¼ oz	9	tr	155
	1 c	12	tr	209
frozen, unsweetened				
heated	½ c sliced	5	tr	48
unheated	½ c sliced	4	tr	41

	Portion	Calcium (mg)	Total Fat (g)	Total Calor
applesauce, canned				
sweetened	½ c	5	tr	97
unsweetened	½ c	4	tr	53
apricots				
raw	3 fruit = 3.7 oz	15	tr	51
canned, w/skin				
in water	3 halves + 1¾ T liquid	7	tr	22
in juice	3 halves + 1¾ T liquid	10	tr	40
in extra light syrup	3 halves + 1¾ T liquid	8	tr	41
in light syrup	3 halves + 1¾ T liquid	10	tr	54
in heavy syrup	3 halves + 1¾ T liquid	7	tr	70
canned, w/out skin				
in water	2 fruit + 2 T liquid	8	tr	20
in heavy syrup	2 fruit + 2 T liquid	8	tr	75
in extra heavy syrup	2 fruit + 2 T liquid	7	tr	87
dehydrated (low-moisture), sulfured				
cooked	½ c	30	tr	156
uncooked	½ c	37	tr	192
dried, sulfured				
cooked, w/added sugar	½ c halves	20	tr	153
cooked, w/out added sugar	½ c halves	20	tr	106
uncooked	10 halves	16	tr	83
frozen, sweetened	½ c	12	tr	119
avocados, raw				
all commercial varieties	1 fruit = 7.1 oz	22	31	324
	1 c puree	25	35	370
California	1 fruit = 6.1 oz	19	30	306
	1 c puree	25	40	407
Florida	1 fruit = 10.7 oz	33	27	339
	1 c puree	25	20	257
bananas				
raw	1 fruit = 4 oz	7	tr	105
dehydrated (banana powder)	1 T	1	tr	21
blackberries				
raw	½ c	23	tr	37
canned, in heavy syrup	½ c	27	tr	118
frozen, unsweetened	1 c	44	1	97

	Portion	Calcium (mg)	Total Fat (g)	Total Calor
blueberries				
raw	1 c	9	1	82
canned, in heavy syrup	½ c	7	tr	112
frozen				
sweetened	1 c	13	tr	187
unsweetened	1 c	12	1	78
boysenberries				
canned, in heavy syrup	½ c	23	tr	113
frozen, unsweetened	1 c	36	tr	66
breadfruit, raw	¼ small fruit = 3.4 oz	17	tr	99
candied fruit *See* BAKING INGREDIENTS				
cantaloupe *See* melons, *below*				
carambolas, raw	1 fruit = 4½ oz	6	tr	42
carissa plums, raw	1 fruit = 0.7 oz	2	tr	12
casaba *See* melons, *below*				
cherimoyas, raw	1 fruit = 19¼ oz	126	2	515
cherries, sour, red				
raw	1 c w/pits	16	tr	51
canned				
in water	½ c	13	tr	43
in light syrup	½ c	13	tr	94
in heavy syrup	½ c	13	tr	116
in extra heavy syrup	½ c	13	tr	148
frozen, unsweetened	1 c	20	1	72
cherries, sweet				
raw	10 fruit = 2.4 oz	10	1	49
canned				
in water	½ c	13	tr	57
in juice	½ c	17	tr	68
in light syrup	½ c	12	tr	85
in heavy syrup	½ c	12	tr	107
in extra heavy syrup	½ c	11	tr	133
frozen, sweetened	1 c	31	tr	232
Chinese gooseberries *See* kiwi fruit, *below*				
coconut *See* BAKING INGREDIENTS; NUTS & NUT-BASED BUTTERS, FLOURS, MEALS, MILKS, PASTES, & POWDERS				
crabapples, raw	1 c sliced	20	tr	83
cranberries, raw	1 c whole	7	tr	46
cranberry sauce, canned, sweetened	½ c	5	tr	209
currants				
European, black, raw	½ c	31	tr	36
red & white, raw	½ c	18	tr	31
zante, dried	½ c	62	tr	204
custard apples, raw	edible portion = 3½ oz	30	1	101

	Portion	Calcium (mg)	Total Fat (g)	Total Calor
dates, domestic, dry	10 fruit = 2.9 oz	27	tr	228
elderberries, raw	1 c	55	1	105
figs				
raw	1 medium fruit = 1¾ oz	18	tr	37
canned				
in water	3 fruit + 1¾ T liquid	22	tr	42
in light syrup	3 fruit + 1¾ T liquid	23	tr	58
in heavy syrup	3 fruit + 1¾ T liquid	23	tr	75
in extra heavy syrup	3 fruit + 1¾ T liquid	22	tr	91
dried				
cooked	½ c	79	1	140
uncooked	10 fruit = 6.6 oz	269	2	477
fruit cocktail, canned				
in water	½ c	6	tr	40
in juice	½ c	10	tr	56
in extra light syrup	½ c	10	tr	55
in light syrup	½ c	8	tr	72
in heavy syrup	½ c	8	tr	93
in extra heavy syrup	½ c	8	tr	115
fruit salad, canned				
in water	½ c	8	tr	37
in juice	½ c	14	tr	62
in light syrup	½ c	8	tr	73
in heavy syrup	½ c	8	tr	94
in extra heavy syrup	½ c	8	tr	114
fruit salad, tropical, canned, in heavy syrup	½ c	17	tr	110
gooseberries				
raw	1 c	38	1	67
canned, in light syrup	½ c	20	tr	93
grandillas *See* passion fruit, *below*				
grapefruit				
raw, pink & red	½ fruit = 4.3 oz	13	tr	37
raw, white	½ fruit = 4.2 oz	14	tr	39
canned				
in water	½ c	18	tr	44
in juice	½ c	19	tr	46
in light syrup	½ c	18	tr	76
grapes				
American type, raw	10 fruit = 0.8 oz	3	tr	15

	Portion	Calcium (mg)	Total Fat (g)	Total Calor
grapes *(cont.)*				
European type, raw	10 fruit = 1.8 oz	5	tr	36
Thompson seedless, canned				
in water	½ c	13	tr	48
in heavy syrup, solids & liquids	½ c	13	tr	94
groundcherries, raw	½ c	6	tr	37
guavas				
common, raw	1 fruit = 3.2 oz	18	1	45
strawberry, raw	1 fruit = 0.2 oz	1	tr	4
guava sauce, cooked	½ c	8	tr	43
honeydew *See* melons, *below*				
jackfruit, raw	edible portion = 3½ oz	34	tr	94
jujubes				
raw	edible portion = 3½ oz	21	tr	79
dried	edible portion = 3½ oz	79	1	287
kiwi fruit, raw	1 medium fruit = 2.7 oz	20	tr	46
kumquats, raw	1 fruit = 0.7 oz	8	tr	12
lemon peel, raw	1 t	3	tr	?
	1 T	8	tr	?
lemons, raw				
w/peel	1 medium fruit = 3.8 oz	66	tr	22
w/out peel	1 medium fruit = 2 oz	15	tr	17
limes, raw	1 fruit = 2.4 oz	22	tr	20
litchis *See* lychees, *below*				
loganberries, frozen	1 c	38	tr	80
longans				
raw	1 fruit = 0.1 oz	0	0	2
dried	edible portion = 3½ oz	45	tr	286
loquats, raw	1 fruit = 0.3 oz	2	tr	5
lychees				
raw	1 fruit = 0.3 oz	0	tr	6
dried	edible portion = 3½ oz	33	1	277

	Portion	Calcium (mg)	Total Fat (g)	Total Calor
mammy apples, raw	1 fruit = 29.8 oz	93	4	431
mangos, raw	1 fruit = 7.3 oz	21	1	135
melon balls, frozen, cantaloupe & honeydew melons	1 c	17	tr	55
cantaloupe, raw	½ fruit = 9.4 oz	28	1	94
	1 c cubed	17	tr	57
casaba, raw	⅒ fruit = 5.8 oz	8	tr	43
	1 c cubed	9	tr	45
honeydew, raw	⅒ fruit = 4½ oz	8	tr	46
	1 c cubed	10	tr	60
muskmelon See cantaloupe, above				
mixed fruit				
canned, in heavy syrup, solids & liquids	½ c	1	tr	92
dried	11 oz	110	1	712
frozen, sweetened	1 c	18	tr	245
mulberries, raw	10 fruit = ½ oz	6	tr	7
muskmelons See melons: cantaloupe, above				
natal plums See carissa plums, above				
nectarines, raw	1 fruit = 4.8 oz	6	1	67
oheloberries, raw	10 fruit = 0.4 oz	1	tr	3
orange peel, raw	1 t	3	0	?
	1 T	10	tr	?
oranges, raw				
w/peel	1 fruit = 5.6 oz	111	tr	64
w/out peel				
all commercial varieties	1 fruit = 4.6 oz	52	tr	62
California, navels	1 fruit = 4.9 oz	56	tr	65
California, Valencias	1 fruit = 4.3 oz	48	tr	59
Florida	1 fruit = 5.3 oz	65	tr	69
papayas, raw	1 fruit = 10.7 oz	72	tr	117
passion fruit, purple, raw	1 fruit = 0.6 oz	2	tr	18
peaches				
raw	1 fruit = 3.1 oz	5	tr	37

	Portion	Calcium (mg)	Total Fat (g)	Total Calor
peaches *(cont.)*				
canned, clingstone				
in water	1 half + 1⅔ T liquid	2	tr	18
in extra light syrup	1 half + 1⅔ T liquid	4	tr	32
in light syrup	1 half + 1¾ T liquid	3	tr	44
canned, clingstone & free-stone				
in juice	1 half + 1⅔ T liquid	5	tr	34
in heavy syrup	1 half + 1¾ T liquid	2	tr	60
canned, freestone, in extra heavy syrup	1 half + 1¾ T liquid	3	tr	77
dehydrated (low-moisture), sulfured				
cooked	½ c	19	1	161
uncooked	½ c	22	1	188
dried, sulfured				
cooked, w/added sugar	½ c halves	11	tr	139
cooked, w/out added sugar	½ c halves	12	tr	99
uncooked	10 halves	37	1	311
frozen, sweetened	1 c sliced, thawed	6	tr	235
peaches, spiced, canned, in heavy syrup	1 fruit + 2 T liquid	5	tr	66
pears				
raw	1 fruit = 5.8 oz	19	1	98
canned				
in water	1 half + 1⅔ T liquid	3	tr	22
in juice	1 half + 1⅔ T liquid	7	tr	38
in extra light syrup	1 half + 1⅔ T liquid	5	tr	36
in light syrup	1 half + 1¾ T liquid	4	tr	45
in heavy syrup	1 half + 1¾ T liquid	4	tr	58
in extra heavy syrup	1 half + 1¾ T liquid	4	tr	77
dried, sulfured				
cooked, w/added sugar	½ c halves	22	tr	196
cooked, w/out added sugar	½ c halves	21	tr	163
uncooked	10 halves	59	1	459
persimmons				
Japanese				
raw	1 fruit = 5.9 oz	13	tr	118

	Portion	Calcium (mg)	Total Fat (g)	Total Calor
dried	1 fruit = 1.2 oz	8	tr	93
native, raw	1 fruit = 0.9 oz	7	tr	32
pineapple				
raw	1 slice = 3 oz	6	tr	42
	1 c diced	11	1	77
canned				
in water	1 slice + 1¼ T liquid	9	tr	19
	1 c tidbits	37	tr	79
in juice	1 slice + 1¼ T liquid	8	tr	35
	1 c chunks or tidbits	34	tr	150
in light syrup	1 slice + 1¼ T liquid	8	tr	30
	1 c	36	tr	131
in heavy syrup	1 slice + 1¼ T liquid	8	tr	45
	1 c chunks, tidbits, or crushed	35	tr	199
in extra heavy syrup	1 slice + 1¼ T liquid	8	tr	48
	1 c chunks or crushed	35	tr	217
frozen, sweetened	½ c chunks	11	tr	104
pitangas, raw	1 fruit = 0.2 oz	1	tr	2
	1 c	16	1	57
plantains				
raw	1 fruit = 6.3 oz	5	1	218
cooked	½ c sliced	2	tr	89
plums, purple				
raw	1 fruit = 2.3 oz	2	tr	36
canned				
in water	3 fruit + 2 T liquid	6	tr	39
	1 c	17	tr	102
in juice	3 fruit + 2 T liquid	9	tr	55
	1 c	25	tr	146
in light syrup	3 fruit + 2¾ T liquid	13	tr	83
	1 c	24	tr	158
in heavy syrup	3 fruit + 2¾ T liquid	12	tr	119
	1 c	24	tr	230

	Portion	Calcium (mg)	Total Fat (g)	Total Calor
plums, purple: canned *(cont.)*				
in extra heavy syrup	3 fruit + 2¾ T liquid	12	tr	135
	1 c	24	tr	265
pomegranates, raw	1 fruit = 5.4 oz	5	tr	104
prickly pears, raw	1 fruit = 3.6 oz	58	1	42
prunes				
canned, in heavy syrup	5 fruit + 2 T liquid	15	tr	90
	1 c	40	tr	245
dehydrated (low-moisture)				
cooked	½ c	34	tr	158
uncooked	½ c	48	tr	224
dried				
cooked, w/added sugar	½ c	25	tr	147
cooked, w/out added sugar	½ c	24	tr	113
uncooked	10 fruit = 3 oz	43	tr	201
	1 c	82	1	385
pummelos, raw	1 fruit = 21.4 oz	23	tr	228
	1 c sections	7	tr	71
quinces, raw	1 fruit = 3.2 oz	10	tr	53
raisins				
golden seedless	1 c not packed	76	1	437
	1 c packed	87	1	498
seeded	1 c not packed	41	1	428
	1 c packed	46	1	488
seedless	1 c not packed	71	1	434
	1 c packed	81	1	494
raspberries, red				
raw	1 c	27	1	61
canned, in heavy syrup, solids & liquids	½ c	14	tr	117
frozen, sweetened	1 c	38	tr	256
	10 oz pkg	43	tr	291
rhubarb				
raw	½ c diced	52	tr	13
frozen				
cooked, w/added sugar	½ c	174	tr	139
uncooked	½ c	132	tr	14
rose apples, raw	edible portion = 3½ oz	29	tr	25
roselles, raw	1 c	123	tr	28

	Portion	Calcium (mg)	Total Fat (g)	Total Calor
sapodillas, raw	1 fruit = 6 oz	36	2	140
sapotes, raw	1 fruit = 7.9 oz	88	1	301
soursops, raw	1 fruit = 22 oz	88	2	416
starfruit *See* carambolas, *above*				
strawberries				
raw	1 c	21	1	45
canned, in heavy syrup	½ c	16	tr	117
frozen, sweetened				
sliced	1 c	28	tr	245
	10 oz pkg	31	tr	273
whole	1 c	29	tr	200
	10 oz pkg	32	tr	223
frozen, unsweetened	1 c	23	tr	52
sugar apples, raw	1 fruit = 5½ oz	37	tr	146
Surinam cherries *See* pitangas, *above*				
sweetsops *See* sugar apples, *above*				
tamarinds, raw	1 fruit = 0.1 oz	1	tr	5
tangerines				
raw	1 fruit = 3 oz	12	tr	37
canned				
in juice, solids & liquids	½ c	14	tr	46
in light syrup, solids & liquids	½ c	9	tr	76
watermelon, raw	¹⁄₁₆ fruit = 17 oz	38	2	152
	1 c diced	13	1	50
West Indian cherries *See* acerolas, *above*				

▪ BRAND NAME

Birds Eye

mixed fruit in syrup	5 oz	<20	0	120
red raspberries in lite syrup	5 oz	20	1	100
strawberries, halved, in lite syrup	5 oz	<20	0	90
strawberries, halved, in syrup	5 oz	<20	0	120

Dole

mandarin oranges in light syrup	½ c	9	tr	76
pineapple cuts in juice	½ c	10	<1	70
pineapple cuts in syrup	½ c	14	tr	95

	Portion	Calcium (mg)	Total Fat (g)	Total Calor
Dromedary				
chopped dates	¼ c	20	0	130
pitted dates	5	20	0	100
Fresh Chef				
Tropical Delight fruit salad	7 oz	60	11	240
Mott's				
applesauce	4 oz	16	0	88
chunky applesauce	4 oz	17	0	57
cinnamon applesauce	4 oz	18	0	72
natural applesauce	4 oz	11	0	44
Mrs. Paul's				
apple fritters	2	20	13	270
Stouffer				
escalloped apples	4 oz	<20	3	140

❑ FRUIT & NUT SNACK MIXES
See SNACKS

❑ FRUIT CHUTNEYS & RELISHES *See*
PICKLES, OLIVES, RELISHES, & CHUTNEYS

❑ FRUIT SAUCES *See* FRUITS, FRESH
& PROCESSED

❑ FRUIT SPREADS

Fruit Butters

apple	1 T	3	tr	37
guava	1 T	?	0	39

Jams

average, all varieties				
regular	1 T	8	tr	55
low-cal	1 T	1	tr	29
grape	1 T	2	tr	59
plum	1 T	2	tr	59

Jellies

average, all varieties				
regular	1 T	4	tr	55
low-cal	1 T	1	0	27

	Portion	Calcium (mg)	Total Fat (g)	Total Calor
blackberry	1 T	4	0	51
boysenberry	1 T	4	0	52
cherry	1 T	3	tr	52
currant	1 T	4	0	52
grape	1 T	4	tr	55
guava	1 T	3	tr	52
quince	1 T	2	tr	51
strawberry	1 T	3	0	51

Marmalades

	Portion	Calcium (mg)	Total Fat (g)	Total Calor
citrus	1 T	7	tr	51
orange	1 T	4	tr	56
papaya	1 T	?	0	57

Preserves

	Portion	Calcium (mg)	Total Fat (g)	Total Calor
apricot	1 T	2	tr	51
apricot-pineapple	1 T	3	tr	51
blackberry	1 T	3	tr	55
boysenberry	1 T	4	tr	54
peach	1 T	2	0	51

▪ BRAND NAME

Smucker's
FRUIT BUTTERS

	Portion	Calcium (mg)	Total Fat (g)	Total Calor
apple	2 t	<20	0	25
peach	2 t	<20	0	30

JAMS, JELLIES, MARMALADES, & PRESERVES

	Portion	Calcium (mg)	Total Fat (g)	Total Calor
all flavors				
regular	2 t	<20	0	35
low-sugar or Slenderella	2 t	<20	0	16
imitation grape jelly or strawberry jam, artificially sweetened	2 t	<20	0	4

❏ GELATIN & GELATIN DESSERTS
See DESSERTS: CUSTARDS, GELATINS, PUDDINGS, & PIE FILLINGS

❏ GRAINS *See* RICE & GRAINS, PLAIN & PREPARED

	Portion	Calcium (mg)	Total Fat (g)	Total Calor

❏ **GRAVIES** *See* SAUCES, GRAVIES, & CONDIMENTS

❏ **HAM** *See* PORK, FRESH & CURED; PROCESSED MEAT & POULTRY PRODUCTS

❏ **HERBS & SPICES** *See* SEASONINGS

❏ **HONEY** *See* SUGARS & SWEETENERS

❏ **HOT DOGS** *See* frankfurter, *under* PROCESSED MEAT & POULTRY PRODUCTS

❏ **ICE CREAM & ICE MILK** *See* DESSERTS, FROZEN

❏ **INFANT & TODDLER FOODS**

Baked Products

	Portion	Calcium (mg)	Total Fat (g)	Total Calor
arrowroot cookies	1	2	1	24
	1 oz	9	4	125
pretzels	1	1	tr	24
	1 oz	7	1	113
teething biscuits	1	29	1	43
	1 oz	75	1	111
zwieback	1	1	1	30
	1 oz	6	3	121

Cereals, Hot & Cold

	Portion	Calcium (mg)	Total Fat (g)	Total Calor
barley				
dry	½ oz	113	tr	52
	1 T	19	tr	9
w/whole milk	1 oz	65	1	31
cereal & egg yolks				
strained	about 4½ oz	30	2	66
	1 oz	7	1	15

	Portion	Calcium (mg)	Total Fat (g)	Total Calor
junior	about 7½ oz	51	4	110
	1 oz	7	1	15
cereal, egg yolks, & bacon				
strained	about 4½ oz	36	7	101
	1 oz	8	1	22
junior	about 7½ oz	54	11	178
	1 oz	7	2	24
grits & egg yolks, strained	about 4½ oz	36	3	?
	1 oz	8	1	?
high protein				
dry	½ oz	103	1	51
	1 T	17	tr	9
w/whole milk	1 oz	62	1	31
high protein w/apple & orange				
dry	½ oz	107	1	53
	1 T	18	tr	9
w/whole milk	1 oz	63	1	32
mixed				
dry	½ oz	104	1	54
	1 T	18	tr	9
w/whole milk	1 oz	62	1	32
mixed w/applesauce & bananas				
strained	about 4.8 oz	9	1	111
	1 oz	2	tr	23
junior	about 7.8 oz	9	1	183
	1 oz	1	tr	24
mixed w/bananas				
dry	½ oz	99	1	56
	1 T	17	tr	9
w/whole milk	1 oz	61	1	33
mixed w/honey				
dry	½ oz	168	1	55
	1 T	28	tr	9
w/whole milk	1 oz	83	1	33
oatmeal				
dry	½ oz	104	1	56
	1 T	18	tr	10
w/whole milk	1 oz	62	1	33
oatmeal w/applesauce & bananas				
strained	about 4.8 oz	11	1	99
	1 oz	2	tr	21
junior	about 7.8 oz	12	2	165
	1 oz	2	tr	21
oatmeal w/bananas				
dry	½ oz	92	1	56
	1 T	16	tr	9
w/whole milk	1 oz	59	1	33

	Portion	Calcium (mg)	Total Fat (g)	Total Calor
oatmeal w/honey				
dry	½ oz	164	1	55
	1 T	28	tr	9
w/whole milk	1 oz	82	1	33
rice				
dry	½ oz	121	1	56
	1 T	20	tr	9
w/whole milk	1 oz	68	1	33
rice w/applesauce & ba-	about 4.8 oz	23	1	107
nanas, strained	1 oz	5	tr	23
rice w/bananas				
dry	½ oz	98	1	57
	1 T	17	tr	10
w/whole milk	1 oz	60	1	33
rice w/honey				
dry	½ oz	166	tr	56
	1 T	28	tr	9
w/whole milk	1 oz	83	1	33
rice w/mixed fruit, junior	about 7.8 oz	43	1	186
	1 oz	6	tr	24

Desserts

	Portion	Calcium (mg)	Total Fat (g)	Total Calor
apple Betty				
strained	about 4.8 oz	25	0	97
	1 oz	5	0	20
junior	about 7.8 oz	36	0	153
	1 oz	5	0	20
caramel pudding				
strained	about 4.8 oz	60	1	104
	1 oz	13	tr	22
junior	about 7½ oz	116	2	167
	1 oz	15	tr	22
cherry vanilla pudding				
strained	about 4.8 oz	7	tr	91
	1 oz	1	tr	19
junior	about 7.8 oz	11	tr	152
	1 oz	1	tr	20
chocolate custard pudding				
strained	about 4½ oz	78	2	107
	1 oz	17	1	24
junior	about 7.8 oz	134	4	195
	1 oz	17	1	25
cottage cheese w/pineapple				
strained	about 4.8 oz	35	1	94
	1 oz	7	tr	20
junior	about 7.8 oz	68	2	172
	1 oz	9	tr	22
Dutch apple				
strained	about 4.8 oz	6	1	92
	1 oz	1	tr	19

	Portion	Calcium (mg)	Total Fat (g)	Total Calor
junior	about 7.8 oz	10	2	151
	1 oz	1	tr	19
fruit dessert				
strained	about 4.8 oz	11	0	79
	1 oz	2	0	17
junior	about 7.8 oz	19	0	138
	1 oz	2	0	18
orange pudding, strained	about 4.8 oz	43	1	108
	1 oz	9	tr	23
peach cobbler				
strained	about 4.8 oz	6	0	88
	1 oz	1	0	18
junior	about 7.8 oz	9	0	147
	1 oz	1	0	19
peach melba				
strained	about 4.8 oz	13	0	81
	1 oz	3	0	17
junior	about 7.8 oz	23	0	132
	1 oz	3	0	17
pineapple orange, strained	about 4½ oz	14	0	89
	1 oz	3	0	20
pineapple pudding				
strained	about 4½ oz	40	tr	104
	1 oz	9	tr	23
junior	about 7.8 oz	75	1	192
	1 oz	10	tr	25
tropical fruit, junior	about 7.8 oz	22	0	131
	1 oz	3	0	17
vanilla custard pudding				
strained	about 4½ oz	71	3	109
	1 oz	16	1	24
junior	about 7.8 oz	123	5	196
	1 oz	16	1	25

Dinners, Regular

	Portion	Calcium (mg)	Total Fat (g)	Total Calor
beef & egg noodles				
strained	about 4½ oz	12	2	68
	1 oz	3	1	15
junior	about 7½ oz	18	4	122
	1 oz	2	1	16
beef & rice, toddler	about 6.2 oz	20	5	146
	1 oz	3	1	23
beef lasagna, toddler	about 6.2 oz	32	4	137
	1 oz	5	1	22
beef stew, toddler	about 6.2 oz	16	2	90
	1 oz	3	tr	14
chicken & noodles				
strained	about 4½ oz	29	2	67
	1 oz	6	tr	15

	Portion	Calcium (mg)	Total Fat (g)	Total Calor
chicken & noodles *(cont.)*				
junior	about 7½ oz	36	3	109
	1 oz	5	tr	15
chicken soup, strained	about 4½ oz	47	2	64
	1 oz	10	1	14
chicken soup, cream of, strained	about 4½ oz	44	2	74
	1 oz	10	1	16
chicken stew, toddler	about 6 oz	60	6	132
	1 oz	10	1	22
lamb & noodles, junior	about 1½ oz	39	5	138
	1 oz	5	1	18
macaroni & bacon, toddler	about 7½ oz	152	7	160
	1 oz	20	1	21
macaroni & cheese				
strained	about 4½ oz	69	3	76
	1 oz	15	1	17
junior	about 7½ oz	108	4	130
	1 oz	14	1	17
macaroni & ham, junior	about 7½ oz	159	3	127
	1 oz	21	tr	17
macaroni, tomato, & beef				
strained	about 4½ oz	21	1	71
	1 oz	5	tr	16
junior	about 7½ oz	30	2	125
	1 oz	4	tr	17
mixed vegetables				
strained	about 4½ oz	29	tr	52
	1 oz	6	0	11
junior	about 7½ oz	37	tr	71
	1 oz	5	0	9
spaghetti, tomato, & meat				
junior	about 7½ oz	39	3	135
	1 oz	5	tr	18
toddler	about 6.2 oz	39	2	133
	1 oz	6	tr	21
split peas & ham, junior	about 7½ oz	49	3	152
	1 oz	7	tr	20
turkey & rice				
strained	about 4½ oz	27	2	63
	1 oz	6	tr	14
junior	about 7½ oz	50	3	104
	1 oz	7	tr	14
vegetables & bacon				
strained	about 4½ oz	17	4	88
	1 oz	4	1	19
junior	about 7½ oz	23	8	150
	1 oz	3	1	20
vegetables & beef				
strained	about 4½ oz	16	3	67
	1 oz	3	1	15

	Portion	Calcium (mg)	Total Fat (g)	Total Calor
junior	about 7½ oz	22	4	113
	1 oz	3	1	15
vegetables & chicken				
strained	about 4½ oz	18	1	55
	1 oz	4	tr	12
junior	about 7½ oz	30	2	106
	1 oz	4	tr	14
vegetables & ham				
strained	about 4½ oz	11	2	62
	1 oz	2	1	14
junior	about 7½ oz	16	4	110
	1 oz	2	1	15
toddler	about 6.2 oz	41	5	128
	1 oz	7	1	21
vegetables & lamb				
strained	about 4½ oz	15	3	67
	1 oz	3	1	15
junior	about 7½ oz	27	4	108
	1 oz	4	1	14
vegetables & liver				
strained	about 4½ oz	9	1	50
	1 oz	2	tr	11
junior	about 7½ oz	20	1	93
	1 oz	3	tr	12
vegetables & turkey				
strained	about 4½ oz	21	2	54
	1 oz	5	tr	12
junior	about 7½ oz	27	3	101
	1 oz	4	tr	13
toddler	about 6.2 oz	82	6	141
	1 oz	13	1	23
vegetables, dumplings, & beef				
strained	about 4½ oz	18	1	61
	1 oz	4	tr	14
junior	about 7½ oz	30	2	103
	1 oz	4	tr	14
vegetables, noodles, & chicken				
strained	about 4½ oz	35	3	81
	1 oz	8	1	18
junior	about 7½ oz	54	5	137
	1 oz	7	1	18
vegetables, noodles, & turkey				
strained	about 4½ oz	41	2	56
	1 oz	9	tr	12
junior	about 7½ oz	67	3	110
	1 oz	9	tr	15

	Portion	Calcium (mg)	Total Fat (g)	Total Calor

Dinners, High in Meat or Cheese

	Portion	Calcium (mg)	Total Fat (g)	Total Calor
beef w/vegetables				
strained	about 4½ oz	15	5	96
	1 oz	3	1	21
junior	about 4½ oz	15	6	108
	1 oz	3	1	24
chicken w/vegetables				
strained	about 4½ oz	66	5	100
	1 oz	15	1	22
junior	about 4½ oz	56	7	117
	1 oz	12	2	26
cottage cheese w/pineapple,	about 4.8 oz	88	3	157
strained	1 oz	18	1	33
ham w/vegetables				
strained	about 4½ oz	14	4	97
	1 oz	3	1	21
junior	about 4½ oz	12	4	98
	1 oz	3	1	22
turkey w/vegetables				
strained	about 4½ oz	80	6	111
	1 oz	18	1	25
junior	about 4½ oz	91	6	115
	1 oz	20	1	25
veal w/vegetables				
strained	about 4½ oz	12	3	89
	1 oz	3	1	20
junior	about 4½ oz	14	4	93
	1 oz	3	1	21

Fruit
See also Desserts, *above*

	Portion	Calcium (mg)	Total Fat (g)	Total Calor
apple blueberry				
strained	about 4.8 oz	5	tr	82
	1 oz	1	tr	17
junior	about 7.8 oz	10	tr	137
	1 oz	1	tr	18
apple raspberry				
strained	about 4.8 oz	7	tr	79
	1 oz	1	0	17
junior	about 7.8 oz	11	tr	127
	1 oz	1	0	16
applesauce				
strained	about 4½ oz	5	tr	53
	1 oz	1	0	12
junior	about 7½ oz	10	0	79
	1 oz	1	0	11
applesauce & apricots				
strained	about 4.8 oz	8	tr	60
	1 oz	2	tr	13

	Portion	Calcium (mg)	Total Fat (g)	Total Calor
junior	about 7.8 oz	13	tr	104
	1 oz	2	tr	13
applesauce & cherries				
strained	about 4.8 oz	14	0	65
	1 oz	3	0	14
junior	about 7.8 oz	20	0	106
	1 oz	3	0	14
applesauce & pineapple				
strained	about 4½ oz	5	tr	48
	1 oz	1	0	11
junior	about 7½ oz	8	tr	83
	1 oz	1	0	11
apricots & tapioca				
strained	about 4.8 oz	12	0	80
	1 oz	3	0	17
junior	about 7.8 oz	18	0	139
	1 oz	2	0	18
bananas & pineapple w/tapioca				
strained	about 4.8 oz	9	tr	91
	1 oz	2	0	19
junior	about 7.8 oz	15	0	143
	1 oz	2	0	18
bananas w/tapioca				
strained	about 4.8 oz	6	tr	77
	1 oz	1	0	16
junior	about 7.8 oz	17	tr	147
	1 oz	2	0	19
guava & papaya w/tapioca, strained	about 4½ oz	9	tr	80
	1 oz	2	0	18
guava w/tapioca, strained	about 4½ oz	9	0	86
	1 oz	2	0	19
mango w/tapioca, strained	about 4.8 oz	5	tr	109
	1 oz	1	tr	23
papaya & applesauce w/tapioca, strained	about 4½ oz	9	tr	89
	1 oz	2	0	20
peaches				
strained	about 4.8 oz	8	tr	96
	1 oz	2	0	20
junior	about 7.8 oz	11	tr	157
	1 oz	1	0	20
pears				
strained	about 4½ oz	11	tr	53
	1 oz	2	0	12
junior	about 7½ oz	18	tr	93
	1 oz	2	0	12
pears & pineapple				
strained	about 4½ oz	13	tr	52
	1 oz	3	0	12

	Portion	Calcium (mg)	Total Fat (g)	Total Calor
pears & pineapple *(cont.)*				
junior	about 7½ oz	21	tr	93
	1 oz	3	tr	12
plums w/tapioca				
strained	about 4.8 oz	8	0	96
	1 oz	2	0	20
junior	about 7.8 oz	12	0	163
	1 oz	2	0	21
prunes w/tapioca				
strained	about 4.8 oz	20	tr	94
	1 oz	4	0	20
junior	about 7.8 oz	33	tr	155
	1 oz	4	0	20

Fruit Juices

	Portion	Calcium (mg)	Total Fat (g)	Total Calor
apple	about 4.2 oz	6	tr	61
	1 fl oz	1	0	14
apple-cherry	about 4.2 oz	7	tr	53
	1 fl oz	2	tr	13
apple-grape	about 4.2 oz	7	tr	60
	1 fl oz	2	tr	14
apple-peach	about 4.2 oz	4	tr	55
	1 fl oz	1	0	13
apple-plum	about 4.2 oz	6	0	63
	1 fl oz	2	0	15
apple-prune	about 4.2 oz	12	tr	94
	1 fl oz	3	0	23
mixed fruit	about 4.2 oz	10	tr	61
	1 fl oz	2	0	14
orange	about 4.2 oz	16	tr	58
	1 fl oz	4	tr	14
orange-apple	about 4.2 oz	13	tr	56
	1 fl oz	3	tr	13
orange-apple-banana	about 4.2 oz	6	tr	61
	1 fl oz	2	0	15
orange-apricot	about 4.2 oz	8	tr	60
	1 fl oz	2	0	14
orange-banana	about 4.2 oz	22	tr	65
	1 fl oz	5	0	15
orange-pineapple	about 4.2 oz	10	tr	63
	1 fl oz	2	0	15
prune-orange	about 4.2 oz	16	tr	91
	1 fl oz	4	tr	22

Meats & Egg Yolks

	Portion	Calcium (mg)	Total Fat (g)	Total Calor
beef				
strained	about 3½ oz	7	5	106
	1 oz	2	2	30

	Portion	Calcium (mg)	Total Fat (g)	Total Calor
junior	about 3½ oz	8	5	105
	1 oz	2	1	30
beef w/beef heart, strained	about 3½ oz	4	4	93
	1 oz	1	1	27
chicken				
strained	about 3½ oz	63	8	128
	1 oz	18	2	37
junior	about 3½ oz	54	10	148
	1 oz	16	3	42
chicken sticks, junior	2½ oz	52	10	134
	1 stick = 0.35 oz	7	1	19
egg yolks, strained	about 3.3 oz	72	16	191
	1 oz	22	5	58
ham				
strained	about 3½ oz	6	6	110
	1 oz	2	2	32
junior	about 3½ oz	5	7	123
	1 oz	1	2	35
lamb				
strained	about 3½ oz	7	5	102
	1 oz	2	1	29
junior	about 3½ oz	7	5	111
	1 oz	2	2	32
liver, strained	about 3½ oz	3	4	100
	1 oz	1	1	29
meat sticks, junior	2½ oz	24	10	130
	1 stick = 0.35 oz	3	2	18
pork, strained	about 3½ oz	5	7	123
	1 oz	1	2	35
turkey				
strained	about 3½ oz	23	6	113
	1 oz	7	2	32
junior	about 3½ oz	28	7	128
	1 oz	8	2	37
turkey sticks, junior	2½ oz	51	10	129
	1 stick = 0.35 oz	7	1	18
veal				
strained	about 3½ oz	7	5	100
	1 oz	2	1	29
junior	about 3½ oz	6	5	109
	1 oz	2	1	31

	Portion	Calcium (mg)	Total Fat (g)	Total Calor
Vegetables				
beans, green				
plain				
strained	about 4½ oz	49	tr	32
	1 oz	11	0	7
junior	about 7.3 oz	133	tr	51
	1 oz	18	0	7
buttered				
strained	about 4½ oz	82	1	42
	1 oz	18	tr	9
junior	about 7.3 oz	143	2	67
	1 oz	20	tr	9
creamed, junior	about 7½ oz	68	1	68
	1 oz	9	tr	9
beets, strained	about 4½ oz	18	tr	43
	1 oz	4	0	10
carrots				
plain				
strained	about 4½ oz	29	tr	34
	1 oz	6	0	8
junior	about 7½ oz	49	tr	67
	1 oz	7	0	9
buttered				
strained	about 4½ oz	45	1	46
	1 oz	10	tr	10
junior	about 7½ oz	76	1	70
	1 oz	10	tr	9
corn, creamed				
strained	about 4½ oz	25	1	73
	1 oz	6	tr	16
junior	about 7½ oz	39	1	138
	1 oz	5	tr	18
garden vegetables, strained	about 4½ oz	36	tr	48
	1 oz	8	tr	11
mixed vegetables				
strained	about 4½ oz	17	1	52
	1 oz	4	tr	11
junior	about 7½ oz	24	1	88
	1 oz	3	tr	12
peas				
plain, strained	about 4½ oz	26	tr	52
	1 oz	6	tr	11
buttered				
strained	about 4½ oz	49	1	72
	1 oz	11	tr	16
junior	about 7.3 oz	93	3	123
	1 oz	13	tr	17
creamed, strained	about 4½ oz	16	2	68
	1 oz	4	1	15

	Portion	Calcium (mg)	Total Fat (g)	Total Calor
spinach, creamed				
strained	about 4½ oz	113	2	48
	1 oz	25	tr	11
junior	about 7½ oz	240	3	90
	1 oz	32	tr	12
squash				
plain				
strained	about 4½ oz	30	tr	30
	1 oz	7	tr	7
junior	about 7½ oz	50	tr	51
	1 oz	7	tr	7
buttered				
strained	about 4½ oz	42	tr	37
	1 oz	9	tr	8
junior	about 7½ oz	65	1	63
	1 oz	9	tr	8
sweet potatoes				
plain				
strained	about 4.8 oz	21	tr	77
	1 oz	4	0	16
junior	about 7.8 oz	35	tr	133
	1 oz	5	0	17
buttered				
strained	about 4.8 oz	28	1	76
	1 oz	6	tr	16
junior	about 7.8 oz	61	2	126
	1 oz	8	tr	16

▪ BRAND NAME

Beech-Nut
STAGE 1

Cereal

barley	½ oz dry	120	0	50
	½ oz dry + 2.4 fl oz milk	210	3	100
oatmeal (calcium-fortified)	½ oz dry	120	1	50
	½ oz dry + 2.4 fl oz milk	210	4	100
rice (calcium-fortified)	½ oz dry	120	1	60
	½ oz dry + 2.4 fl oz milk	210	3	100

Fruit & Fruit Dishes

bartlett pears	4½ oz	12	0	70
Chiquita bananas	4½ oz	<12	0	100

	Portion	Calcium (mg)	Total Fat (g)	Total Calor
golden delicious applesauce	4½ oz	<12	0	60
yellow cling peaches	4½ oz	<12	0	60
Fruit Juices				
apple	4.2 fl oz	<12	0	60
pear	4.2 fl oz	12	0	60
white grape	4.2 fl oz	12	0	80
Meat				
beef	3½ oz	<12	8	120
chicken	3½ oz	36	6	110
lamb	3½ oz	<12	8	130
turkey	3½ oz	24	7	120
veal	3½ oz	<12	7	120
Vegetables				
butternut squash	4½ oz	24	0	40
green beans	4½ oz	60	0	40
regal imperial carrots	4½ oz	24	0	40
sweet potatoes	4½ oz	24	0	70
tender sweet peas	4½ oz	24	0	70
STAGE 2				
Cereals				
Hi-Protein (calcium-fortified)	½ oz dry	120	1	50
	½ oz dry + 2.4 fl oz milk	180	3	90
mixed (calcium-fortified)	½ oz dry	120	1	50
	½ oz dry + 2.4 fl oz milk	210	3	100
w/applesauce & bananas oatmeal	4½ oz	12	0	80
w/applesauce & bananas	4½ oz	12	1	90
w/bananas (calcium-fortified)	½ oz dry	90	1	60
	½ oz dry + 2.4 fl oz milk	180	3	100
rice				
w/applesauce & bananas	4½ oz	36	0	100
w/bananas (calcium-fortified)	½ oz dry	90	0	60
	½ oz dry + 2.4 fl oz milk	180	3	100
Desserts				
banana custard	4½ oz	48	1	120
banana pineapple	4½ oz	<12	0	100

	Portion	Calcium (mg)	Total Fat (g)	Total Calor
Dutch apple	4½ oz	12	0	80
guava tropical fruit	4½ oz	<12	0	100
mango tropical fruit	4½ oz	<12	0	90
papaya tropical fruit	4½ oz	<12	0	80
vanilla custard	4½ oz	60	3	130
Fruit & Dairy				
cottage cheese w/pineapple	4½ oz	24	1	110
mixed fruit & yogurt	4½ oz	36	1	110
peaches & yogurt	4½ oz	36	1	110
Fruit & Fruit Dishes				
apples & grapes	4½ oz	<12	0	90
apples & strawberries	4½ oz	<12	0	90
applesauce & apricots	4½ oz	<12	0	60
applesauce & bananas	4½ oz	<12	0	60
applesauce & cherries	4½ oz	<12	0	70
apples, mandarin oranges, & bananas	4½ oz	<12	0	90
apples, peaches, & strawberries	4½ oz	<12	0	100
apples, pears, & bananas	4½ oz	<12	0	90
apricots w/pears & applesauce	4½ oz	12	0	70
bananas w/pears & applesauce	4½ oz	<12	0	90
bartlett pears & pineapple	4½ oz	24	0	70
Fruit Dessert	4½ oz	<12	0	80
Island Fruits	4½ oz	<12	0	90
pears & applesauce	4½ oz	<12	0	70
plums w/rice	4½ oz	<12	0	110
prunes w/pears	4½ oz	24	0	120
Juice				
Juice Plus	4 fl oz	12	0	80
Main Courses				
beef & egg noodles w/vegetables	4½ oz	12	4	90
Beef Dinner Supreme	4½ oz	12	7	120
chicken & rice w/vegetables	4½ oz	12	3	80
chicken noodle w/vegetables	4½ oz	24	3	90
macaroni, tomato, & beef	4½ oz	24	3	90
Turkey Dinner Supreme	4½ oz	36	5	110
turkey rice w/vegetables	4½ oz	24	2	70
vegetable beef	4½ oz	12	3	90
vegetable chicken	4½ oz	60	3	90
vegetable ham	4½ oz	12	3	90

	Portion	Calcium (mg)	Total Fat (g)	Total Calor
vegetable lamb	4½ oz	12	3	90
Vegetables				
creamed corn	4½ oz	12	0	90
garden vegetables	4½ oz	24	0	60
mixed vegetables	4½ oz	12	0	50
peas & carrots	4½ oz	36	0	60
STAGE 3				
Custard				
banana	7½ oz	60	2	200
vanilla	7½ oz	120	5	210
Fruit & Dairy				
cottage cheese w/pineapple	7½ oz	36	2	190
mixed fruit & yogurt	7½ oz	60	1	170
peaches & yogurt	7½ oz	60	2	190
Fruit & Fruit Dishes				
apples & grapes	7½ oz	<12	0	190
apples & strawberries	7½ oz	12	0	160
applesauce	7½ oz	12	0	100
applesauce & bananas	7½ oz	12	0	110
applesauce & cherries	7½ oz	12	0	110
apples, mandarin oranges, & bananas	7½ oz	12	0	150
apples, peaches, & strawberries	7½ oz	12	0	160
apples, pears, & bananas	7½ oz	12	0	160
apricots w/pears & apples	7½ oz	24	0	120
bananas w/pears & apples	7½ oz	12	0	160
bartlett pears	7½ oz	24	0	110
bartlett pears & pineapple	7½ oz	36	0	120
Fruit Dessert	7½ oz	<12	0	130
Island Fruits	7½ oz	<12	0	150
peaches	7½ oz	<12	0	150
Main Courses & Dinners				
beef & egg noodles w/vegetables	7½ oz	24	5	150
Beef Dinner Supreme	7½ oz	24	9	180
chicken noodles w/vegetables	7½ oz	24	4	140
macaroni, tomato, & beef	7½ oz	24	5	150
spaghetti, tomato, & beef	7½ oz	36	5	170
Turkey Dinner Supreme	7½ oz	60	8	190
turkey rice w/vegetables	7½ oz	36	4	130
vegetable bacon	7½ oz	24	9	180
vegetable beef	7½ oz	24	5	150
vegetable chicken	7½ oz	60	5	140

	Portion	Calcium (mg)	Total Fat (g)	Total Calor
vegetable lamb	7½ oz	12	5	140
Vegetables				
carrots	7½ oz	48	0	60
green beans	7½ oz	90	0	60
mixed vegetables	7½ oz	24	0	90
sweet potatoes	7½ oz	26	0	120
UNSTAGED				
Juices				
apple	4 fl oz	<12	0	60
apple banana	4.2 fl oz	<12	0	60
apple cherry	4.2 fl oz	<12	0	50
apple cranberry	4.2 fl oz	<12	0	60
apple grape	4.2 fl oz	<12	0	60
apple pear	4.2 fl oz	12	0	60
mixed fruit	4.2 fl oz	<12	0	60
orange	4.2 fl oz	12	0	60
pear	4 fl oz	12	0	60
tropical blend	4 fl oz	12	0	70
TABLE TIME				
Main Courses				
beef stew	6 oz	24	4	140
pasta squares in meat sauce	6 oz	24	4	140
spaghetti rings in meat sauce	6 oz	36	4	160
vegetable stew w/chicken	6 oz	36	8	190
Soups				
Hearty chicken w/stars	6 oz	24	9	180
Hearty vegetable	6 oz	12	0	70
Gerber				
BAKED GOODS				
all	1 serving	<16	?	50– 60
CHUNKY PRODUCTS				
beef & egg noodles w/vegetables	6 oz	16	4	130
Homestyle noodles & beef	6 oz	32	6	150
macaroni alphabets w/beef & tomato sauce	6¼ oz	16	3	130
noodles & chicken w/carrots & peas	6 oz	16	2	100
potatoes & ham	6 oz	16	4	110
rice w/beef & tomato sauce	6¼ oz	16	5	150
saucy rice w/chicken	6 oz	32	2	110
spaghetti tomato sauce & beef	6¼ oz	48	5	160
vegetables & beef	6¼ oz	16	5	140

	Portion	Calcium (mg)	Total Fat (g)	Total Calor
vegetables & chicken	6¼ oz	16	5	140
vegetables & ham	6¼ oz	16	4	120
vegetables & turkey	6¼ oz	48	3	110

DRY CEREALS, READY-TO-SERVE

barley	½ oz dry	90	1	60
	½ oz dry + 2.4 fl oz milk	180	4	110
high protein	½ oz dry	90	1	50
	½ oz dry + 2.4 fl oz milk	180	4	100
w/apple & orange	½ oz dry	90	1	60
	½ oz dry + 2.4 fl oz milk	180	4	100
mixed	½ oz dry	90	1	50
	½ oz dry + 2.4 fl oz milk	180	4	100
w/banana	½ oz dry	90	1	60
	½ oz dry + 2.4 fl oz milk	180	4	100
oatmeal	½ oz dry	90	1	50
	½ oz dry + 2.4 fl oz milk	180	4	100
w/banana	½ oz dry	90	1	60
	½ oz dry + 2.4 fl oz milk	180	4	100
rice	½ oz dry	90	1	60
	½ oz dry + 2.4 fl oz milk	180	4	100
w/banana	½ oz dry	90	1	60
	½ oz dry + 2.4 fl oz milk	180	4	100

STRAINED FOODS

Cereals w/Fruit

mixed w/applesauce & bananas	4½ oz	<12	1	100
oatmeal w/applesauce & bananas	4½ oz	<12	1	100
rice w/applesauce & bananas	4½ oz	12	1	100

	Portion	Calcium (mg)	Total Fat (g)	Total Calor
Desserts				
banana apple	4½ oz	<12	1	90
cherry vanilla pudding	4½ oz	<12	1	90
chocolate custard pudding	4½ oz	60	2	110
Dutch apple	4½ oz	<12	2	100
fruit	4½ oz	<12	1	100
Hawaiian Delight	4½ oz	48	1	120
orange pudding	4½ oz	48	1	110
peach cobbler	4½ oz	<12	1	100
vanilla custard pudding	4½ oz	60	1	100
Dinners, Regular				
beef egg noodle	4½ oz	<12	3	90
cereal egg yolk bacon	4½ oz	48	5	100
chicken noodle	4½ oz	24	2	80
cream of chicken soup	4½ oz	36	2	70
macaroni cheese	4½ oz	60	3	90
macaroni tomato beef	4½ oz	12	2	80
turkey rice	4½ oz	12	3	80
vegetable bacon	4½ oz	12	5	100
vegetable beef	4½ oz	<12	3	80
vegetable chicken	4½ oz	12	2	80
vegetable ham	4½ oz	<12	3	80
vegetable lamb	4½ oz	12	4	90
vegetable liver	4½ oz	<12	1	60
vegetable turkey	4½ oz	12	2	70
Dinners, High in Meat				
beef w/vegetables	4½ oz	<12	6	120
chicken w/vegetables	4½ oz	48	8	140
ham w/vegetables	4½ oz	<12	4	100
turkey w/vegetables	4½ oz	12	7	130
veal w/vegetables	4½ oz	<12	4	100
Fruit & Tropical Fruit				
apple blueberry	4½ oz	<12	1	60
applesauce	4½ oz	<12	0	60
applesauce apricot	4½ oz	<12	1	70
applesauce w/pineapple	4½ oz	<12	1	60
apricots w/tapioca	4½ oz	<12	1	90
bananas w/pineapple & tapioca	4½ oz	<12	1	70
bananas w/tapioca	4½ oz	<12	0	100
guava w/tapioca	4½ oz	<12	1	90
mango w/tapioca	4½ oz	<12	1	90
papaya w/tapioca	4½ oz	<12	1	80
peaches	4½ oz	<12	1	90
pear pineapple	4½ oz	12	1	80
pears	4½ oz	12	1	80

	Portion	Calcium (mg)	Total Fat (g)	Total Calor
plums w/tapioca	4½ oz	<12	1	100
prunes w/tapioca	4½ oz	12	1	100
Tropical Fruit Medley	4½ oz	<12	1	80
Juices				
apple	4.2 oz	<12	0	60
apple apricot	4.2 oz	<12	0	60
apple banana	4.2 oz	<12	1	70
apple cherry	4.2 oz	<12	0	60
apple grape	4.2 oz	<12	0	60
apple peach	4.2 oz	<12	0	60
apple pineapple	4.2 oz	<12	0	60
apple plum	4.2 oz	<12	0	60
apple prune	4.2 oz	12	0	70
mixed fruit	4.2 oz	12	1	70
orange	4.2 oz	12	1	70
orange apple	4.2 oz	12	1	70
pear	4.2 oz	12	0	60
Meats & Egg Yolks				
beef	3½ oz	<12	5	100
beef liver	3½ oz	<12	4	100
chicken	3½ oz	<12	9	140
egg yolks	3½ oz	24	17	190
ham	3½ oz	60	6	110
lamb	3½ oz	<12	5	100
pork	3½ oz	<12	6	110
turkey	3½ oz	<12	8	130
veal	3½ oz	<12	5	100
Vegetables				
beets	4½ oz	12	0	50
carrots	4½ oz	24	1	40
creamed corn	4½ oz	24	1	80
creamed spinach	4½ oz	120	1	60
garden vegetables	4½ oz	36	1	50
green beans	4½ oz	48	1	50
mixed vegetables	4½ oz	12	1	50
peas	4½ oz	24	1	60
squash	4½ oz	24	1	40
sweet potatoes	4½ oz	12	1	80
FIRST FOODS				
Fruit				
applesauce	2½ oz	<12	0	30
bananas	2½ oz	<12	0	60
peaches	2½ oz	<12	0	30
pears	2½ oz	<12	0	40

	Portion	Calcium (mg)	Total Fat (g)	Total Calor
Vegetables				
carrots	2½ oz	12	1	30
green beans	2½ oz	24	0	20
peas	2½ oz	<12	1	40
squash	2½ oz	<12	0	20
sweet potatoes	2½ oz	<12	0	50
JUNIOR FOODS				
Cereals w/Fruit				
mixed w/applesauce & bananas	7½ oz	12	2	170
oatmeal w/applesauce & bananas	7½ oz	12	2	160
rice w/mixed fruit	7½ oz	36	1	170
Desserts				
banana apple	7½ oz	<12	1	150
cherry vanilla pudding	7½ oz	<12	1	150
Dutch apple	7½ oz	<12	2	160
fruit	7½ oz	12	1	160
Hawaiian Delight	7½ oz	90	1	190
peach cobbler	7½ oz	<12	1	160
vanilla custard pudding	7½ oz	120	2	190
Dinners, Regular				
beef egg noodle	7½ oz	12	4	140
chicken noodle	7½ oz	24	3	120
macaroni tomato beef	7½ oz	12	3	130
spaghetti tomato sauce beef	7½ oz	24	2	140
split peas ham	7½ oz	36	3	150
turkey rice	7½ oz	24	4	120
vegetable bacon	7½ oz	36	8	180
vegetable beef	7½ oz	24	4	140
vegetable chicken	7½ oz	36	3	120
vegetable ham	7½ oz	12	4	140
vegetable lamb	7½ oz	12	5	140
vegetable turkey	7½ oz	12	3	120
Dinners, High in Meat				
beef w/vegetables	4½ oz	12	7	130
chicken w/vegetables	4½ oz	48	7	130
ham w/vegetables	4½ oz	<12	4	110
turkey w/vegetables	4½ oz	12	8	140
veal w/vegetables	4½ oz	<12	4	110
Fruit				
apple blueberry	7½ oz	<12	1	110
applesauce	7½ oz	<12	1	100

	Portion	Calcium (mg)	Total Fat (g)	Total Calor
applesauce apricot	7½ oz	<12	1	110
apricots w/tapioca	7½ oz	12	1	160
bananas w/pineapple & tapioca	7½ oz	12	1	110
bananas w/tapioca	7½ oz	<12	0	160
peaches	7½ oz	<12	1	140
pear pineapple	7½ oz	12	1	120
pears	7½ oz	12	1	120
plums w/tapioca	7½ oz	12	1	160
Meats				
beef	3½ oz	<12	5	110
chicken	3½ oz	24	9	140
ham	3½ oz	<12	7	120
lamb	3½ oz	<12	5	100
turkey	3½ oz	<12	8	130
veal	3½ oz	<12	5	100
Vegetables				
carrots	7½ oz	48	1	60
creamed corn	7½ oz	36	1	130
creamed green beans	7½ oz	60	1	100
mixed vegetables	7½ oz	24	1	90
peas	7½ oz	36	1	110
squash	7½ oz	48	1	70
sweet potatoes	7½ oz	24	1	140
TODDLER FOODS				
Cereals				
Toasted Oat Rings	½ oz dry	120	1	60
	½ oz dry + 2.7 fl oz milk	200	4	110
Juices				
all	4 oz	<16	0	60
Meat & Poultry Sticks				
chicken	2½ oz	32	8	120
meat	2½ oz	32	7	110
turkey	2½ oz	64	9	120
Health Valley				
instant brown rice cereal	½ oz or 2 T	3	1	60
sprouted cereal w/bananas	½ oz or 2 T	11	1	50
Nabisco				
zwieback teething toast	2	<20	1	60

❑ **JAMS & JELLIES** *See* FRUIT SPREADS

	Portion	Calcium (mg)	Total Fat (g)	Total Calor

❑ **JUICE, FROZEN** *See* DESSERTS, FROZEN

❑ **JUICES & JUICE DRINKS**
See BEVERAGES

❑ **LAMB, VEAL, & MISCELLANEOUS MEATS**

Lamb, Cooked

	Portion	Calcium (mg)	Total Fat (g)	Total Calor
lamb chops (3/lb w/bone)				
lean & fat				
arm, braised	2.2 oz	16	15	220
loin, broiled	2.8 oz	16	16	235
rib	3½ oz	8	37	423
lean only				
arm, braised	1.7 oz	12	7	135
loin, broiled	2.3 oz	12	6	140
leg of lamb, roasted				
lean & fat	3 oz	8	13	205
lean only	2.6 oz	6	6	140
rib, roasted				
lean & fat	3 oz	19	26	315
lean only	2 oz	12	7	130

Veal, Cooked

	Portion	Calcium (mg)	Total Fat (g)	Total Calor
arm steak, lean & fat	3½ oz	10	19	298
blade, lean & fat	3½ oz	11	17	276
breast, stewed w/gravy	2.6 oz	8	19	256
cutlet, medium fat, bone removed				
braised or broiled	3 oz	9	9	185
breaded	3½ oz	0	15	319
flank, medium fat, stewed	3½ oz	11	32	390
foreshank, medium fat, stewed	3½ oz	12	10	216
loin chop, lean & fat	3½ oz	6	36	421
plate, medium fat, stewed	3½ oz	12	21	303
rib, roasted	3 oz	10	14	230

Other Meats

	Portion	Calcium (mg)	Total Fat (g)	Total Calor
alligator, raw	3½ oz	1,231	4	232
armadillo, raw	3½ oz	30	5	172

	Portion	Calcium (mg)	Total Fat (g)	Total Calor
frog legs				
raw	4 large	18	tr	73
flour-coated & fried	6 large	28	29	418
goat, raw	3½ oz	11	9	165
guinea pig, raw	3½ oz	29	2	96
hare, raw	3½ oz	12	5	135
rabbit, stewed	3½ oz	21	10	216
venison, roasted	3½ oz	20	2	146
whale meat, raw	3½ oz	12	8	156

❑ LEGUMES & LEGUME PRODUCTS

Beans

	Portion	Calcium (mg)	Total Fat (g)	Total Calor
adzuki				
boiled	½ c	32	tr	147
canned, sweetened	½ c	33	tr	351
yokan (sugar & bean confection)	1½ oz	4	tr	36
black, boiled	½ c	24	tr	113
black turtle soup				
boiled	1 c	103	1	241
canned	½ c	42	tr	109
broad				
raw	½ c	77	1	256
boiled	½ c	31	tr	93
canned, solids & liquids	½ c	34	tr	91
cannellini *See* kidney, *below*				
cranberry				
boiled	½ c	44	tr	120
canned, solids & liquids	½ c	44	tr	108
fava *See* broad, *above*				
French, boiled	½ c	54	1	111
garbanzo *See* chickpeas, *under* Peas & Lentils, *below*				
great northern				
boiled	½ c	60	tr	104
canned, solids & liquids	½ c	69	1	150
green gram *See* mung, *below*				
hyacinth, boiled	½ c	39	1	114
kidney				
all types				
boiled	½ c	25	tr	112
canned, solids & liquids	½ c	35	tr	104
California red, boiled	½ c	58	tr	109
red				
boiled	½ c	25	tr	112
canned, solids & liquids	½ c	31	tr	108
royal red, boiled	½ c	39	tr	108

	Portion	Calcium (mg)	Total Fat (g)	Total Calor
lima				
baby				
boiled	½ c	26	tr	115
frozen, boiled, drained	10 oz pkg	89	1	326
	½ c	25	tr	94
large				
boiled	½ c	16	tr	108
canned, solids & liquids	½ c	25	tr	95
frozen, boiled, drained	10 oz pkg	67	1	312
	½ c	19	tr	85
long rice See mung, *below*				
lupins, boiled	½ c	42	2	98
miso See fermented products, *under* SOYBEANS & SOYBEAN PRODUCTS				
moth, boiled	½ c	3	tr	103
mung				
boiled	½ c	27	tr	107
mature seeds, sprouted				
raw	½ c	7	tr	16
	12 oz pkg	43	1	102
boiled, drained	½ c	7	tr	13
canned, drained	½ c	9	tr	8
stir-fried	½ c	8	tr	31
long rice, dehydrated, prepared from mung bean starch	½ c	17	tr	246
mungo, boiled	½ c	48	tr	95
natto See fermented products, *under* SOYBEANS & SOYBEAN PRODUCTS				
navy, canned, solids & liquids	½ c	62	1	148
okara See tofu: okara, *under* SOYBEANS & SOYBEAN PRODUCTS				
pink, boiled	½ c	44	tr	125
pinto				
boiled	½ c	41	tr	117
canned, solids & liquids	½ c	44	tr	93
frozen, boiled, drained	10 oz pkg	149	1	460
Roman See cranberry, *above*				
shellie See beans, shellie, *under* VEGETABLES, PLAIN & PREPARED				
small white, boiled	½ c	66	1	127
snap See beans, snap, *under* VEGETABLES, PLAIN & PREPARED				
soybeans See SOYBEANS & SOYBEAN PRODUCTS				
tempeh See fermented products, *under* SOYBEANS & SOYBEAN PRODUCTS				
white				
boiled	½ c	81	tr	125
canned, solids & liquids	½ c	96	tr	153
winged				
raw	½ c	400	15	372
boiled	½ c	122	5	126
winged bean leaves, raw	3½ oz	224	1	74
winged bean tuber, raw	3½ oz	30	1	159
yardlong				
raw	½ c	116	1	292
boiled	½ c	36	tr	102

	Portion	Calcium (mg)	Total Fat (g)	Total Calor
yellow, boiled	½ c	55	1	126
yokan *See* adzuki, *above*				

Peas & Lentils

	Portion	Calcium (mg)	Total Fat (g)	Total Calor
Bengal gram *See* chickpeas, *below*				
black-eyed *See* cowpeas, common, *below*				
chickpeas				
boiled	½ c	40	2	134
canned, solids & liquids	½ c	39	1	143
cowpeas, catjang, boiled	½ c	22	1	100
cowpeas, common				
boiled	½ c	21	tr	100
canned, plain, solids & liquids	½ c	24	1	92
cowpeas, leafy tips				
raw	1 c	23	tr	10
boiled, drained	½ c	18	tr	6
cowpeas, young pods w/ seeds				
raw	1 pod = 0.4 oz	8	tr	5
boiled, drained	½ c	26	tr	16
crowder peas *See* cowpeas, common, *above*				
golden gram *See* chickpeas, *above*				
lentils				
boiled	½ c	19	tr	115
sprouted				
raw	½ c	9	tr	40
stir-fried	3½ oz	14	tr	101
pigeon peas				
raw	½ c	133	2	350
boiled	½ c	36	tr	102
red gram *See* pigeon peas, *above*				
southern peas *See* cowpeas, common, *above*				
split peas, boiled	½ c	13	tr	116

Prepared Bean Dishes

	Portion	Calcium (mg)	Total Fat (g)	Total Calor
baked beans				
canned				
plain or vegetarian	½ c	64	1	118
w/beef	½ c	60	5	161
w/franks	½ c	61	8	182
w/pork	½ c	66	2	133
w/pork & sweet sauce	½ c	77	2	140
w/pork & tomato sauce	½ c	70	1	123
homemade	½ c	77	6	190
chili w/beans, canned	½ c	60	7	144

	Portion	Calcium (mg)	Total Fat (g)	Total Calor
cowpeas, common, canned, w/pork	½ c	21	2	99
falafel	0.6 oz	9	3	57
	1.8 oz	27	9	170
hummus	1 c	124	21	420
refried beans, canned	½ c	59	1	134

▪ BRAND NAME

Arrowhead Mills
adzuki beans	2 oz	60	1	190
anasazi beans	2 oz	80	1	200
black turtle beans	2 oz	80	1	190
chickpeas	2 oz	80	3	200
kidney beans	2 oz	60	1	190
lentils				
green	2 oz	40	1	190
red	2 oz	40	1	195
mung beans				
dry, raw	2 oz	60	?	?
sprouted	1 c	?	0	50
pinto beans	2 oz	80	1	200
split peas, green	2 oz	20	1	200

Campbell
barbecue beans	7⅞ oz	80	4	250
Home Style beans	8 oz	100	4	270
Old Fashioned beans in molasses & brown sugar	8 oz	100	3	270
pork & beans in tomato sauce	8 oz	80	3	240
Ranchero beans	7⅞ oz	80	5	220

Fearn
BEAN MIXES
bean barley stew	½ of 3½ oz box	20	2	180
black bean Creole	½ of 3¾ oz box	40	2	180
lentil minestrone soup	½ of 3¾ oz box	40	1	160
split pea soup	½ of 3½ oz box	40	3	180
tri-bean casserole	½ of 3¼ oz box	40	2	160

VEGETARIAN MIXES
breakfast patty	⅛ of 7.4 oz box	40	6	110
falafel	⅑ of 7.4 oz box	40	2	80

	Portion	Calcium (mg)	Total Fat (g)	Total Calor
sesame burger	¼ c dry or ⅛ of 8.4 oz box	40	7	130
sunflower burger	¼ c dry or ⅛ of 8.4 oz box	40	4	120

Health Valley
BEANS

Boston baked, regular or no salt	4 oz	22	1	130
vegetarian, w/miso	4 oz	53	1	120

CHILI

con carne	4 oz	43	8	170
mild vegetarian w/beans				
regular	4 oz	3	7	170
no salt	4 oz	20	7	170
spicy vegetarian w/beans				
regular	4 oz	3	7	170
no salt	4 oz	3	7	180
w/lentils, regular or low-sodium	4 oz	40	6	120

LENTILS

Zesty pilaf				
regular	4 oz	44	3	110
no salt	4 oz	33	3	110

Joan of Arc Canned Vegetables

blackeye peas	½ c	20	<1	90
butter beans	½ c	40	<1	100
chili beans	½ c	20	1	100
garbanzo beans	½ c	40	1	90
great northern beans	½ c	60	<1	90
kidney beans				
dark red	½ c	40	<1	110
light red	½ c	40	<1	90
navy beans	½ c	60	<1	100
pinto beans	½ c	60	<1	100
pork & beans	½ c	60	<1	130
small red beans	½ c	40	<1	100

Van Camp's

Beanee Weenee	1 c	95	15	326
brown sugar beans	1 c	121	5	284
butter beans	1 c	41	1	162
chili				
w/beans	1 c	63	23	352
w/out beans	1 c	46	34	412
kidney beans				
dark red	1 c	52	1	182

	Portion	Calcium (mg)	Total Fat (g)	Total Calor
light red	1 c	55	1	184
New Orleans–style red	1 c	59	1	178
Mexican-style chili beans	1 c	75	2	210
pork & beans	1 c	97	2	216
red beans	1 c	84	1	194
vegetarian-style beans	1 c	93	1	206
Western-style beans	1 c	73	4	207
Wolf				
chili w/beans	1 c	59	22	345
chili w/out beans				
regular	1 c	64	27	387
extra spicy	scant c	60	25	363

❑ **LUNCHEON MEATS** *See* PROCESSED MEAT & POULTRY PRODUCTS

❑ **MAIN COURSES** *See* ENTREES & MAIN COURSES, CANNED & BOXED; ENTREES & MAIN COURSES, FROZEN

❑ **MARGARINE** *See* BUTTER & MARGARINE SPREADS

❑ **MARMALADE** *See* FRUIT SPREADS

❑ **MAYONNAISE** *See* SALAD DRESSINGS, MAYONNAISE, VINEGAR, & DIPS

❑ **MEAT** *See* BEEF, FRESH & CURED; LAMB, VEAL, & MISCELLANEOUS MEATS; PORK, FRESH & CURED; PROCESSED MEAT & POULTRY PRODUCTS

❑ **MEAT PRODUCTS, SIMULATED** *See* LEGUMES & LEGUME PRODUCTS; NUTS & NUT-BASED BUTTERS, FLOURS, MEALS, MILKS, PASTES, & POWDERS; SOYBEANS & SOYBEAN PRODUCTS

	Portion	Calcium (mg)	Total Fat (g)	Total Calor

❑ **MEAT SPREADS** *See* PROCESSED MEAT
& POULTRY PRODUCTS

❑ **MILK, MILK SUBSTITUTES, & MILK PRODUCTS: CREAM, SOUR CREAM, CREAM SUBSTITUTES, MILK, MILK SUBSTITUTES, WHEY, & YOGURT**
See also Flavored Milk Beverages, *under*
BEVERAGES; CHEESE & CHEESE FOODS; DESSERT
SAUCES, SYRUPS, & TOPPINGS

Cream & Sour Cream

CREAM

	Portion	Calcium (mg)	Total Fat (g)	Total Calor
half & half	1 T	16	2	20
	1 c	254	28	315
light	1 T	14	3	29
	1 c	231	46	469
medium (25% fat)	1 T	14	4	37
	1 c	216	60	583
whipping				
light	1 T	10	5	44
	1 c or about 2 c whipped	166	74	699
heavy	1 T	10	6	52
	1 c or about 2 c whipped	154	88	821

SOUR CREAM

	Portion	Calcium (mg)	Total Fat (g)	Total Calor
cultured	1 T	14	3	26
	1 c	268	48	493
half & half, cultured	1 T	16	2	20

Cream & Sour Cream Substitutes

coffee whitener, nondairy	Portion	Calcium (mg)	Total Fat (g)	Total Calor
liquid, frozen	½ fl oz	1	2	20
	½ c	11	12	163
liquid, frozen, containing lauric acid oil & sodium caseinate	½ fl oz	1	2	20
	½ c	11	12	164
powdered, containing lauric acid oil & sodium casein-ate	1 t	tr	1	11

	Portion	Calcium (mg)	Total Fat (g)	Total Calor
imitation sour cream, non-dairy, cultured, containing lauric acid oil & sodium caseinate	1 oz	1	6	59
	1 c	6	45	479
sour dressing, nonbutterfat, cultured (made by combining fats or oils other than milk fat w/milk solids)	1 T	14	2	21
	1 c	266	39	417

Milk, Cows'

FRESH

whole

3.7% fat, pasteurized or raw	1 c	290	9	157
low-sodium	1 c	246	8	149

low-fat

2% fat	1 c	297	5	121
2% fat, nonfat milk solids added	1 c	313	5	125
2% fat, protein-fortified	1 c	352	5	137
1% fat	1 c	300	3	102
1% fat, nonfat milk solids added	1 c	313	2	104
1% fat, protein-fortified	1 c	349	3	119
skim	1 c	302	tr	86
skim, nonfat milk solids added	1 c	316	1	90
skim, protein-fortified	1 c	352	1	100
buttermilk, cultured	1 c	285	2	99

CONDENSED & EVAPORATED

condensed, sweetened, canned	1 oz	108	3	123
	1 c	868	27	982

evaporated, canned

whole	1 oz	82	2	42
	½ c	329	10	169
skim	1 fl oz	92	tr	25
	½ c	369	tr	99

DRY

whole	¼ c	292	9	159
	1 c	1,168	34	635

nonfat

regular	¼ c	377	tr	109
	1 c	1,508	1	435
calcium-reduced	1 oz	79	tr	100

	Portion	Calcium (mg)	Total Fat (g)	Total Calor
nonfat *(cont.)*				
instant	3.2 oz	1,120	1	326
	1 c	837	tr	244
buttermilk, sweet cream	1 T	77	tr	25
	1 c	1,421	7	464

Milk, Other

goat	1 c	326	10	168
human	1 oz	10	1	21
Indian buffalo	1 c	412	17	236
sheep	1 c	474	17	264

Milk Substitutes

filled (made by blending hydrogenated vegetable oils w/milk solids)	1 c	312	8	154
filled, w/lauric acid oil (made by combining milk solids w/fats or oils other than milk fat)	1 c	312	8	153
imitation, containing blend of hydrogenated vegetable oils	1 c	79	8	150
imitation, containing lauric acid	1 c	79	8	150

Whey

acid				
dry	1 T	59	tr	10
fluid	1 c	253	tr	59
sweet				
dry	1 T	59	tr	26
fluid	1 c	115	1	66

Yogurt

plain				
8 g protein	1 c	274	7	139
low-fat, 12 g protein	1 c	415	4	144
skim milk, 13 g protein	1 c	452	tr	127
coffee & vanilla varieties, low-fat, 11 g protein	1 c	389	3	194
fruit varieties, low-fat				
9 g protein	1 c	314	3	225
10 g protein	1 c	345	2	231
11 g protein	1 c	383	3	239

	Portion	Calcium (mg)	Total Fat (g)	Total Calor
▪ BRAND NAME				
Colombo Yogurt				
LITE				
plain	8 oz	400	0	110
strawberry	8 oz	300	0	200
vanilla	8 oz	400	0	160
WHOLE MILK				
plain	8 oz	350	7	150
banana strawberry	8 oz	250	6	235
blueberry	8 oz	250	7	250
French vanilla	8 oz	300	7	210
peach	8 oz	250	6	230
strawberry	8 oz	250	6	230
strawberry vanilla	8 oz	250	6	260
Friendship				
buttermilk, low-fat (1½% milk fat)	1 c	300	4	120
Lite Delite low-fat sour cream	2 T	40	2	35
sour cream	2 T	80	5	55
yogurt				
regular (3½% milk fat), plain	1 c	400	8	170
low-fat (1½% milk fat)				
vanilla & coffee	1 c	400	3	210
w/fruit	1 c	350	3	230
Land O'Lakes				
buttermilk	8 fl oz	300	2	100
Flash instant, nonfat, reconstituted dry milk	8 fl oz	300	<1	80
Gourmet heavy whipping cream	1 T	<20	6	60
half & half	1 T	<20	2	20
milk				
homogenized	8 fl oz	300	8	150
low-fat (2%)	8 fl oz	300	5	120
low-fat (1%)	8 fl oz	300	3	100
skim	8 fl oz	300	<1	90
sour cream	1 T	<20	3	25
whipping cream	1 T	<20	5	45
La Yogurt				
plain	6 oz	250	3	130
Rich's Nondairy Creamers				
Coffee Rich	½ oz	tr	2	22
Poly Rich	½ oz	tr	1	22
Richwhip				
liquid	¼ oz or 1 fl oz whipped	tr	2	20

	Portion	Calcium (mg)	Total Fat (g)	Total Calor
Richwhip *(cont.)*				
pressurized	¼ oz	tr	2	20
prewhipped	1 T whipped	tr	1	12
Whitney's Yogurt				
plain	6 oz	350	7	150
apples & raisins	6 oz	250	5	200
blueberry	6 oz	250	5	200
boysenberry	6 oz	250	5	200
cherry	6 oz	250	5	200
coffee	6 oz	300	6	200
lemon	6 oz	300	6	200
peach	6 oz	250	5	200
piña colada	6 oz	250	7	210
raspberry	6 oz	250	5	200
strawberry	6 oz	250	5	200
strawberry banana	6 oz	250	5	200
tropical fruits	6 oz	250	6	200
vanilla	6 oz	300	6	200
wild berries	6 oz	250	5	200

❑ MOLASSES *See* SUGARS & SWEETENERS

❑ MUFFINS *See* BREADS, ROLLS, BISCUITS, & MUFFINS

❑ NOODLES & PASTA, PLAIN

Noodles

	Portion	Calcium (mg)	Total Fat (g)	Total Calor
chow mein, canned	1 c	14	11	220
egg, enriched, cooked	1 c	16	2	200
Japanese style, seasoned *See* Nissin, *under* SOUPS, PREPARED				

Pasta

	Portion	Calcium (mg)	Total Fat (g)	Total Calor
macaroni, enriched, cooked (cut lengths, elbows, shells)				
firm stage, hot	1 c	14	1	190
tender stage				
cold	1 c	8	tr	115
hot	1 c	11	1	155

	Portion	Calcium (mg)	Total Fat (g)	Total Calor
prepared & seasoned pasta dishes *See* DINNERS, FROZEN; ENTREES & MAIN COURSES, CANNED & BOXED; ENTREES & MAIN COURSES, FROZEN				
spaghetti, enriched, cooked				
firm stage, hot	1 c	14	1	190
tender stage, hot	1 c	11	1	155

• BRAND NAME

Health Valley

	Portion	Calcium (mg)	Total Fat (g)	Total Calor
elbows, whole-wheat or whole-wheat w/4 vegetables	2 oz dry	20	1	202
lasagna, whole-wheat	2 oz dry	20	1	200
spaghetti: whole-wheat, whole-wheat amaranth, or whole-wheat w/spinach	2 oz dry	20	1	200
spinach lasagna, whole-wheat	2 oz dry	20	1	170
Mueller's				
egg noodles	2 oz dry	20	3	220
Golden Rich egg noodles	2 oz dry	20	3	220
lasagna	2 oz dry	<20	1	210
spaghetti & macaroni	2 oz dry	<20	1	210
tricolor twists	2 oz dry	<20	1	210
Prince				
egg noodles	3½ oz uncooked	17	3	380
macaroni & spaghetti	3½ oz uncooked	14	2	370
Superoni	3½ oz uncooked	26	0	360

❑ NUTS & NUT-BASED BUTTERS, FLOURS, MEALS, MILKS, PASTES, & POWDERS
See also SEEDS & SEED-BASED BUTTERS, FLOURS, & MEALS

	Portion	Calcium (mg)	Total Fat (g)	Total Calor
acorn flour, full-fat	1 oz	12	9	142
acorns				
raw	1 oz	12	7	105
dried	1 oz	15	9	145
almond butter				
plain	1 T	43	9	101
honey & cinnamon	1 T	43	8	96
almond meal, partially defatted	1 oz	120	5	116

	Portion	Calcium (mg)	Total Fat (g)	Total Calor
almond paste	1 oz	65	8	127
	1 c firmly packed	523	62	1,012
almond powder				
full-fat	1 oz	62	15	168
	1 c not packed	142	34	385
partially defatted	1 oz	67	5	112
	1 c not packed	154	10	255
almonds				
dried				
blanched	1 oz	70	15	166
	1 c whole kernels	358	76	850
unblanched	1 oz	75	15	167
	1 c whole kernels	377	74	837
dry roasted, unblanched	1 oz	80	15	167
	1 c whole kernels	389	71	810
oil roasted				
blanched	1 oz	55	16	174
	1 c whole kernels	276	80	870
unblanched	1 oz	66	16	176
	1 c whole kernels	367	91	970
toasted, unblanched	1 oz	80	14	167
beechnuts, dried	1 oz	0	14	164
Brazil nuts, dried, un-blanched	1 oz	50	19	186
	1 c	246	93	919
butternuts, dried	1 oz	15	16	174
cashew butter, plain	1 T	7	8	94
cashew nuts				
dry roasted	1 oz	13	13	163
	1 c wholes & halves	62	64	787
oil roasted	1 oz	12	14	163
	1 c wholes & halves	53	63	748
chestnuts, Chinese				
raw	1 oz	5	tr	64
boiled, steamed	1 oz	3	tr	44
dried	1 oz	8	1	103
roasted	1 oz	5	tr	68
chestnuts, European				
raw				
peeled	1 oz	5	tr	56
unpeeled	1 oz	8	1	60
	1 c	40	3	308
boiled, steamed	1 oz	13	tr	37

	Portion	Calcium (mg)	Total Fat (g)	Total Calor
dried				
peeled	1 oz	18	1	105
unpeeled	1 oz	19	1	106
roasted	1 oz	8	1	70
	1 c	42	3	350
chestnuts, Japanese				
raw	1 oz	9	tr	44
boiled, steamed	1 oz	3	tr	16
dried	1 oz	20	tr	102
	1 c	111	2	558
roasted	1 oz	10	tr	57
coconut cream				
raw	1 T	2	5	49
	1 c	26	83	792
canned	1 T	0	3	36
	1 c	4	52	568
coconut meat				
raw	1.6 oz	6	15	159
	1 c shredded or grated	12	27	283
dried (desiccated)				
creamed	1 oz	7	20	194
sweetened, flaked, canned	4 oz	16	36	505
	1 c	11	24	341
sweetened, flaked, packaged	7 oz	28	64	944
	1 c	10	24	351
sweetened, shredded	7 oz	30	71	997
	1 c	14	33	466
toasted	1 oz	8	13	168
unsweetened	1 oz	7	18	187
coconut milk				
raw	1 T	2	4	35
	1 c	39	57	552
canned	1 T	3	3	30
	1 c	40	48	445
frozen	1 T	1	3	30
	1 c	11	50	486
coconut water	1 T	4	tr	3
	1 c	58	tr	46
filberts or hazelnuts				
dried				
blanched	1 oz	55	19	191
unblanched	1 oz	53	18	179
	1 c chopped kernels	216	72	727
dry roasted, unblanched	1 oz	55	19	188
oil roasted, unblanched	1 oz	56	18	187
formulated nuts, wheat-based				
unflavored	1 oz	7	16	177
macadamia-flavored	1 oz	6	16	176
all other flavors	1 oz	6	18	184

	Portion	Calcium (mg)	Total Fat (g)	Total Calor
ginkgo nuts				
raw	1 oz	1	tr	52
canned	1 oz	1	tr	32
	1 c	6	3	173
dried	1 oz	6	1	99
hazelnuts See filberts, *above*				
hickory nuts, dried	1 oz	17	18	187
macadamia nuts				
dried	1 oz	20	21	199
	1 c	94	99	940
oil roasted	1 oz	1	22	204
	1 c wholes or halves	2	103	962
mixed nuts (cashew nuts, almonds, filberts, & pecans)				
dry roasted, w/peanuts	1 oz	20	15	169
	1 c	96	70	814
oil roasted				
w/peanuts	1 oz	31	16	175
	1 c	153	80	876
w/out peanuts	1 oz	30	16	175
	1 c	153	81	886
peanut butter, w/added fat, sugar, & salt				
chunk style	2 T	13	16	188
smooth style	2 T	11	16	188
peanut flour				
defatted	1 T	6	tr	13
	1 c	84	tr	196
low-fat	1 c	78	13	257
peanuts				
all types				
raw	1 oz	26	14	159
	1 c	134	72	828
boiled	½ c	18	7	102
dried	1 oz	17	14	161
	1 c	85	72	827
dry roasted	1 oz	15	14	164
	1 c	79	73	855
oil roasted	1 oz	25	14	163
	1 c	126	71	837
Spanish, oil roasted	1 oz	28	14	162
	1 c	147	72	851
Valencia, oil roasted	1 oz	15	14	165
	1 c	78	74	848
Virginia, oil roasted	1 oz	24	14	161
	1 c	123	70	826
pecan flour	1 oz	9	tr	93

	Portion	Calcium (mg)	Total Fat (g)	Total Calor
pecans				
dried	1 oz	10	19	190
	1 c halves	39	73	721
dry roasted	1 oz	10	18	187
oil roasted	1 oz	10	20	195
	1 c	37	78	754
pignolias *See* pine nuts, *below*				
pili nuts, dried	1 oz	41	23	204
	1 c	174	95	863
pine nuts				
pignolia, dried	1 oz	7	14	146
	1 T	3	5	51
piñon, dried	1 oz	2	17	161
	10 kernels	0	1	6
pistachios				
dried	1 oz	38	14	164
	1 c	173	62	739
dry roasted	1 oz	20	15	172
	1 c	90	68	776
sweet chestnuts *See* chestnuts, European, *above*				
walnuts				
black, dried	1 oz	16	16	172
	1 c chopped	72	71	759
English or Persian, dried	1 oz	27	18	182
	1 c pieces	113	74	770

• BRAND NAME

Arrowhead Mills				
peanut butter, creamy or chunky	2 T	<20	16	190
Blue Diamond				
almonds				
raw, whole, unblanched	1 oz	80	14	173
blanched, sliced	1 oz	72	15	176
dry roasted, unsalted	1 oz	92	15	168
oil roasted, salted	1 oz	87	16	174
hazelnuts				
raw, whole, Oregon	1 oz	40	15	166
oil roasted, salted	1 oz	51	18	180
macadamia nuts, dry roasted, salted	1 oz	21	21	193
pistachios, dry roasted, salted, natural, California	1 oz	41	14	162
Erewhon				
almond butter	1 T	28	8	90
peanut butter				
chunky or creamy, salted	2 T	21	14	190
chunky or creamy, unsalted	2 T	7	14	190

	Portion	Calcium (mg)	Total Fat (g)	Total Calor
Fearn				
Brazil nut burger mix	¼ c dry or ⅛ of 7.6 oz box	60	4	100
Planters				
almonds				
blanched: slivered, whole, or sliced	1 oz	60	15	170
dry roasted	1 oz	80	15	170
honey roasted	1 oz	40	13	170
cashews				
dry roasted, regular or unsalted	1 oz	<20	13	230
honey roasted	1 oz	<20	12	170
oil roasted, fancy or halves, regular or unsalted	1 oz	<20	14	170
cashews & peanuts, honey roasted	1 oz	<20	12	170
mixed nuts				
dry roasted				
regular	1 oz	20	14	160
unsalted	1 oz	20	15	170
oil roasted				
deluxe	1 oz	20	17	180
regular or unsalted	1 oz	20	16	180
nut topping	1 oz	<20	16	180
peanuts				
cocktail, oil roasted, regular or unsalted	1 oz	<20	15	170
dry roasted				
regular	1 oz	<20	14	160
unsalted	1 oz	<20	15	170
honey roasted				
regular	1 oz	<20	13	170
dry roasted	1 oz	<20	13	160
oil roasted, salted	1 oz	<20	15	170
redskin, oil roasted	1 oz	<20	15	170
roasted-in-shell, salted or unsalted	1 oz	20	14	160
Spanish				
raw	1 oz	<20	12	150
dry roasted	1 oz	<20	14	160
oil roasted	1 oz	<20	15	170
Sweet 'n Crunchy	1 oz	20	8	140
pecans: chips, halves, or pieces	1 oz	20	20	190
pistachios				
dry roasted	1 oz	20	15	170
natural	1 oz	20	5	170
red	1 oz	20	15	170

	Portion	Calcium (mg)	Total Fat (g)	Total Calor
sesame nut mix				
dry roasted	1 oz	<20	12	160
oil roasted	1 oz	20	13	160
sunflower nuts				
dry roasted				
regular	1 oz	20	14	160
unsalted	1 oz	20	15	170
oil roasted	1 oz	20	15	170
Tavern Nuts	1 oz	<20	15	170
walnuts				
black	1 oz	20	17	180
English: whole, halves, or pieces	1 oz	20	20	190
Skippy Peanut Butter				
creamy or super chunk	2 T	<20	17	190
	1 T	<20	8	95
Smucker's				
natural peanut butter	2 T	0	16	200

❑ **OILS** *See* FATS, OILS, & SHORTENINGS

❑ **OLIVES** *See* PICKLES, OLIVES, RELISHES, & CHUTNEYS

❑ **PASTA** *See* NOODLES & PASTA, PLAIN

❑ **PASTRIES** *See* DESSERTS: CAKES, PASTRIES, & PIES

❑ **PÂTÉS** *See* PROCESSED MEAT & POULTRY PRODUCTS

❑ **PEANUT BUTTER** *See* NUTS & NUT-BASED BUTTERS, FLOURS, MEALS, MILKS, PASTES, & POWDERS

❑ **PICKLES, OLIVES, RELISHES, & CHUTNEYS**
See also peppers; sauerkraut, *under* VEGETABLES, PLAIN & PREPARED

	Portion	Calcium (mg)	Total Fat (g)	Total Calor
Chutneys				
apple	1 T	5	tr	41
tomato	1 T	5	?	31
Olives, Canned				
green	4 medium or 3 extra large	8	2	15
ripe, Mission, pitted	3 small or 2 large	10	2	15
Pickles, Cucumber				
bread & butter	4 slices	8	tr	18
dill, whole	1 medium = about 2¼ oz	17	tr	5
fresh-pack	2 slices = about ½ oz	5	tr	10
kosher	1	7	tr	7
sour	1 large	17	tr	10
sweet	1 large	12	tr	146
sweet & sour, sliced	1 slice	7	tr	3
sweet gherkin, small, whole	1 = about ½ oz	2	tr	20
Relishes				
cranberry-orange	1 T	3	tr	27
canned	½ c	15	tr	246
pickle				
chow chow				
sour	1 oz	9	tr	8
sweet	1 oz	6	tr	32
sour	1 T	4	tr	3
sweet, finely chopped	1 T	3	tr	20
strawberry	1 T	3	0	53
strawberry-pineapple	1 T	3	0	54
tomato	1 T	2	tr	53
• **BRAND NAME**				
Claussen				
bread & butter pickle slices	1	4	0	4
kosher pickle slices	1	1	0	1
kosher tomatoes	1	4	tr	5

	Portion	Calcium (mg)	Total Fat (g)	Total Calor
kosher whole pickles	1	8	tr	7
no-garlic dills	1	19	tr	12
pickle relish	1 T	16	tr	13
sweet pickles	1	8	tr	30
Dromedary				
pimientos, all types, drained	1 oz	<20	0	10
Vlasic				
pickled cucumbers, onions, or peppers	1 oz	<20	0	varies
relishes, hamburger or hot dog	1 oz	<20	0	varies

❑ PIE FILLINGS *See* DESSERTS: CUSTARDS, GELATINS, PUDDINGS, & PIE FILLINGS

❑ PIES *See* DESSERTS: CAKES, PASTRIES, & PIES

❑ PIZZA

	Portion	Calcium (mg)	Total Fat (g)	Total Calor
pizza, cheese	⅛ pizza (15″ diam)	220	9	290

▪ BRAND NAME

	Portion	Calcium (mg)	Total Fat (g)	Total Calor
Celentano				
9-slice pizza	⅑ pizza = 2.67 oz	60	5	157
thick crust pizza	⅓ pizza = 4.3 oz	90	7	238
Celeste Frozen Pizza				
Canadian-style bacon	7¾ oz pizza	491	26	541
	¼ of 19 oz pizza	301	17	329
cheese	6½ oz pizza	375	25	497
	¼ of 17¾ oz pizza	204	17	317
deluxe	8¼ oz pizza	332	32	582
	¼ of 22¼ oz pizza	267	22	378
pepperoni	6¾ oz pizza	336	30	546
	¼ of 19 oz pizza	186	21	368

	Portion	Calcium (mg)	Total Fat (g)	Total Calor
sausage	7½ oz pizza	371	32	571
	¼ of 20 oz pizza	322	22	376
sausage & mushroom	8½ oz pizza	362	32	592
	¼ of 22½ oz pizza	310	22	387
Suprema	9 oz pizza	454	39	678
	¼ of 23 oz pizza	295	24	381
Pepperidge Farm Croissant Pastry Pizza				
cheese	1	400	27	490
deluxe	1	350	27	520
hamburger	1	150	27	510
pepperoni	1	300	25	490
sausage	1	350	29	540
Stouffer's French Bread Frozen Pizza				
cheese	½ pkg	200	13	340
deluxe	½ pkg	200	21	430
hamburger	½ pkg	200	18	410
pepperoni	½ pkg	200	18	390
sausage	½ pkg	200	20	420
sausage & mushroom	½ pkg	100	17	400

❑ PORK, FRESH & CURED
See also PROCESSED MEAT & POULTRY PRODUCTS

Pork, Fresh

retail cuts, separable fat, cooked	1 oz	1	21	200

LEG (HAM)
Lean & Fat

whole, roasted	3 oz	5	18	250
	1 c	9	29	411
rump half, roasted	3 oz	6	15	233
	1 c	10	25	384
shank half, roasted	3 oz	5	19	258
	1 c	9	31	425

Lean Only

whole, roasted	3 oz	6	9	187
	1 c	10	15	309
rump half, roasted	3 oz	6	9	187
	1 c	10	15	309
shank half, roasted	3 oz	6	9	183
	1 c	10	15	301

	Portion	Calcium (mg)	Total Fat (g)	Total Calor
LOIN, WHOLE				
Lean & Fat				
braised	3 oz	7	24	312
	1 chop (3 chops/lb as purchased)	6	20	261
broiled	3 oz	6	23	294
	1 chop (3 chops/lb as purchased)	5	22	284
roasted	3 oz	7	21	271
	1 chop (3 chops/lb as purchased)	7	20	262
Lean Only				
braised	3 oz	8	12	232
	1 chop (3 chops/lb as purchased)	5	8	150
broiled	3 oz	6	13	218
	1 chop (3 chops/lb as purchased)	5	10	169
roasted	3 oz	7	12	204
	1 chop (3 chops/lb as purchased)	6	10	166
LOIN, BLADE				
Lean & Fat				
braised	3 oz	12	29	348
	1 chop (3 chops/lb as purchased)	9	23	275
broiled	3 oz	9	29	334
	1 chop (3 chops/lb as purchased)	8	26	303
pan-fried	3 oz	8	31	352
	1 chop (3 chops/lb as purchased)	9	33	368
roasted	3 oz	10	26	310
	1 chop (3 chops/lb as purchased)	11	27	321

	Portion	Calcium (mg)	Total Fat (g)	Total Calor
Lean Only				
braised	3 oz	14	18	266
	1 chop (3 chops/lb as purchased)	9	10	156
broiled	3 oz	11	18	255
	1 chop (3 chops/lb as purchased)	8	13	177
pan-fried	3 oz	11	17	240
	1 chop (3 chops/lb as purchased)	8	12	175
roasted	3 oz	12	16	238
	1 chop (3 chops/lb as purchased)	10	14	198
LOIN, CENTER				
Lean & Fat				
braised	3 oz	5	22	301
	1 chop (3 chops/lb as purchased)	4	19	266
broiled	3 oz	4	19	269
	1 chop (3 chops/lb as purchased)	4	19	275
pan-fried	3 oz	4	26	318
	1 chop (3 chops/lb as purchased)	4	27	333
roasted	3 oz	5	18	259
	1 chop (3 chops/lb as purchased)	5	19	268
Lean Only				
braised	3 oz	5	12	231
	1 chop (3 chops/lb as purchased)	4	8	166
broiled	3 oz	4	9	196
	1 chop (3 chops/lb as purchased)	3	8	166

	Portion	Calcium (mg)	Total Fat (g)	Total Calor
pan-fried	3 oz	4	14	226
	1 chop (3 chops/lb as purchased)	3	11	178
roasted	3 oz	5	11	204
	1 chop (3 chops/lb as purchased)	4	10	180

LOIN, CENTER RIB
Lean & Fat

	Portion	Calcium (mg)	Total Fat (g)	Total Calor
braised	3 oz	9	23	312
	1 chop (3 chops/lb as purchased)	7	18	246
broiled	3 oz	11	22	291
	1 chop (3 chops/lb as purchased)	10	20	264
pan-fried	3 oz	6	28	331
	1 chop (3 chops/lb as purchased)	6	29	343
roasted	3 oz	8	20	271
	1 chop (3 chops/lb as purchased)	8	19	252

Lean Only

	Portion	Calcium (mg)	Total Fat (g)	Total Calor
braised	3 oz	10	12	236
	1 chop (3 chops/lb as purchased)	6	8	147
broiled	3 oz	13	13	219
	1 chop (3 chops/lb as purchased)	9	9	162
pan-fried	3 oz	7	13	219
	1 chop (3 chops/lb as purchased)	5	9	160
roasted	3 oz	9	12	208
	1 chop (3 chops/lb as purchased)	7	9	162

	Portion	Calcium (mg)	Total Fat (g)	Total Calor
LOIN, SIRLOIN				
Lean & Fat				
braised	3 oz	5	22	299
	1 chop (3 chops/lb as purchased)	5	18	250
broiled	3 oz	4	21	281
	1 chop (3 chops/lb as purchased)	4	21	278
roasted	3 oz	8	17	247
	1 chop (3 chops/lb as purchased)	8	17	244
Lean Only				
braised	3 oz	6	11	221
	1 chop (3 chops/lb as purchased)	4	7	149
broiled	3 oz	5	12	207
	1 chop (3 chops/lb as purchased)	4	9	165
roasted	3 oz	8	11	201
	1 chop (3 chops/lb as purchased)	7	10	175
LOIN, TENDERLOIN				
lean, roasted	3 oz	7	4	141
LOIN, TOP				
Lean & Fat				
braised	3 oz	9	25	324
	1 chop (3 chops/lb as purchased)	7	20	267
broiled	3 oz	10	24	306
	1 chop (3 chops/lb as purchased)	10	23	295
pan-fried	3 oz	6	28	333
	1 chop (3 chops/lb as purchased)	6	29	337

	Portion	Calcium (mg)	Total Fat (g)	Total Calor
roasted	3 oz	8	21	280
	1 chop (3 chops/lb as purchased)	8	21	274
Lean Only				
braised	3 oz	10	12	236
	1 chop (3 chops/lb as purchased)	6	8	147
broiled	3 oz	13	13	219
	1 chop (3 chops/lb as purchased)	9	10	165
pan-fried	3 oz	7	13	219
	1 chop (3 chops/lb as purchased)	5	9	157
roasted	3 oz	9	12	208
	1 chop (3 chops/lb as purchased)	7	9	167
SHOULDER, WHOLE				
lean & fat, roasted	3 oz	6	22	277
	1 c	10	36	456
lean only, roasted	3 oz	6	13	207
	1 c	11	21	341
SHOULDER, ARM PICNIC				
Lean & Fat				
braised	3 oz	6	22	293
	1 c	10	36	483
roasted	3 oz	6	22	281
	1 c	11	37	463
Lean Only				
braised	3 oz	7	10	211
	1 c	12	17	347
roasted	3 oz	7	11	194
	1 c	12	18	319
SHOULDER, BLADE, BOSTON				
Lean & Fat				
braised	3 oz	6	24	316
	1 steak	11	46	594
broiled	3 oz	5	24	297
	1 steak	10	53	647
roasted	3 oz	6	21	273
	1 steak	12	47	594

	Portion	Calcium (mg)	Total Fat (g)	Total Calor
Lean Only				
braised	3 oz	6	15	250
	1 steak	10	23	382
broiled	3 oz	5	16	233
	1 steak	9	28	413
roasted	3 oz	6	14	218
	1 steak	11	27	404
SPARERIBS				
lean & fat, braised	3 oz	40	26	338
	6¼ oz (yield from 1 lb as purchased)	83	54	703
VARIETY MEATS				
brains, braised	3 oz	8	8	117
chitterlings, simmered	3 oz	23	24	258
ears, simmered	1	20	12	183
feet, simmered	2½ oz	32	9	138
heart, braised	1	9	7	191
kidneys, braised	1 c	18	7	211
liver, braised	3 oz	9	4	141
lungs, braised	3 oz	7	3	84
tail, simmered	3 oz	12	30	336
tongue, braised	3 oz	16	16	230
Pork, Cured				
bacon, pan-fried or roasted	3 medium slices (20 slices/lb)	2	9	109
breakfast strips, cooked	3 slices (15 slices/12 oz)	5	12	156
	6 oz	24	62	780
Canadian-style bacon, un-heated, fully cooked as purchased	2 oz	5	4	89
feet, pickled	1 oz	9	5	58
ham, boneless				
regular (about 11% fat)				
unheated	1 oz	2	3	52
	1 c	10	15	255
roasted	3 oz	7	8	151
	1 c	12	13	249
extra lean (about 5% fat)				
unheated	1 oz	2	1	37
	1 c	10	7	183
roasted	3 oz	7	5	123
	1 c	11	8	203

	Portion	Calcium (mg)	Total Fat (g)	Total Calor
ham, canned				
regular (about 13% fat)				
unheated	1 oz	2	4	54
	1 c	8	18	266
roasted	3 oz	7	13	192
	1 c	12	21	317
extra lean (about 4% fat)				
unheated	1 oz	2	1	34
	1 c	8	6	168
roasted	3 oz	5	4	116
	1 c	8	7	191
ham, center slice				
Country Style, lean only, raw	4 oz	?	9	220
	1 oz	?	2	55
lean & fat, unheated, fully	4 oz	8	15	229
cooked as purchased	1 oz	2	4	57
ham patties				
unheated, fully cooked as purchased	2.3 oz	5	18	206
grilled	2 oz	5	18	203
ham steak, boneless, extra lean, unheated, fully cooked as purchased	2 oz	2	2	69
ham, whole				
lean & fat				
unheated, fully cooked as	1 oz	2	5	70
purchased	1 c	10	26	345
roasted	3 oz	6	14	207
	1 c	10	23	341
lean only				
unheated, fully cooked as	1 oz	2	2	42
purchased	1 c	10	8	206
roasted	3 oz	6	5	133
	1 c	10	8	219
salt pork, raw	1 oz	2	23	212
separable fat (from ham & arm picnic)				
unheated, fully cooked as purchased	1 oz	1	17	164
roasted	1 oz	2	18	167
shoulder				
arm picnic, roasted				
lean & fat	3 oz	9	18	238
	1 c	14	30	392
lean only	3 oz	9	6	145
	1 c	15	10	238
blade roll, lean & fat				
unheated, fully cooked as purchased	1 oz	2	6	76
roasted	3 oz	6	20	244

	Portion	Calcium (mg)	Total Fat (g)	Total Calor

- ## BRAND NAME

Armour & Armour Star

	Portion	Calcium (mg)	Total Fat (g)	Total Calor
ham, boneless, cooked, lower salt, 93% fat-free	1 oz	<20	1	35
ham, Speedy Cut, boneless, cooked	1 oz	<20	3	44

Oscar Mayer

	Portion	Calcium (mg)	Total Fat (g)	Total Calor
all bacon, cooked	1 slice	<2	1–6	varies
breakfast strips, raw	1 strip	1	5	52
all sliced ham	1 oz	<3	1–4	varies

❑ POULTRY, FRESH & PROCESSED

See also PROCESSED MEAT & POULTRY PRODUCTS

NOTE: Values are based on the following weights as purchased with giblets & neck:

chicken	
broilers or fryers	3.33 lbs
roasting	4.56 lbs
stewing	2.93 lbs
capons	6.5 lbs

duck	
domesticated	4.42 lbs
wild	2.26 lbs
goose	8.25 lbs
guinea	1.92 lbs
pheasant	2.15 lbs
quail	0.27 lb
squab	0.67 lb

turkey	
all classes	15.47 lbs
fryer-roasters	7.05 lbs
young hens	12.54 lbs
young toms	23.06 lbs

Chicken, Fresh

CHICKEN, BROILERS OR FRYERS

flesh, skin, giblets, & neck	Portion	Calcium (mg)	Total Fat (g)	Total Calor
fried				
batter-dipped	1 chicken	218	180	2,987
flour-coated	1 chicken	123	108	1,928

	Portion	Calcium (mg)	Total Fat (g)	Total Calor
roasted	1 chicken	105	90	1,598
stewed	1 chicken	104	93	1,625
flesh & skin				
fried				
batter-dipped	½ chicken	97	81	1,347
flour-coated	½ chicken	52	47	844
roasted	½ chicken	45	41	715
stewed	½ chicken	44	42	730
flesh only				
fried	1 c	24	13	307
roasted	1 c	21	10	266
stewed	1 c	19	9	248
skin only				
fried				
batter-dipped	½ chicken	49	55	748
flour-coated	½ chicken	8	24	281
roasted	½ chicken	8	23	254
stewed	½ chicken	9	24	261
giblets				
fried, flour-coated	1 c	26	20	402
simmered	1 c	18	7	228
gizzard, simmered	1 c	14	5	222
heart, simmered	1 c	27	11	268
liver, simmered	1 c	20	8	219
light meat w/skin				
fried				
batter-dipped	½ chicken	37	29	520
flour-coated	½ chicken	20	16	320
roasted	½ chicken	19	14	293
stewed	½ chicken	19	15	302
dark meat w/skin				
fried				
batter-dipped	½ chicken	59	52	828
flour-coated	½ chicken	32	31	523
roasted	½ chicken	25	26	423
stewed	½ chicken	25	27	428
light meat w/out skin				
fried	1 c	22	8	268
roasted	1 c	21	6	242
stewed	1 c	18	6	223
dark meat w/out skin				
fried	1 c	25	16	334
roasted	1 c	21	14	286
stewed	1 c	20	13	269
back, meat & skin				
fried				
batter-dipped	½ back	31	26	397
flour-coated	½ back	17	15	238
roasted	½ back	11	11	159
stewed	½ back	11	11	158

	Portion	Calcium (mg)	Total Fat (g)	Total Calor
back, meat only				
fried	½ back	15	9	167
roasted	½ back	10	5	96
stewed	½ back	9	5	88
breast, meat & skin				
fried				
batter-dipped	½ breast	28	18	364
flour-coated	½ breast	16	9	218
roasted	½ breast	14	8	193
stewed	½ breast	14	8	202
breast, meat only				
fried	½ breast	14	4	161
roasted	½ breast	13	3	142
stewed	½ breast	12	3	144
drumstick, meat & skin				
fried				
batter-dipped	1	12	11	193
flour-coated	1	6	7	120
roasted	1	6	6	112
stewed	1	7	6	116
drumstick, meat only				
fried	1	5	3	82
roasted	1	5	2	76
stewed	1	5	3	78
leg (drumstick & thigh), meat & skin				
fried				
batter-dipped	1	28	26	431
flour-coated	1	15	16	285
roasted	1	14	15	265
stewed	1	14	16	275
leg (drumstick & thigh), meat only				
fried	1	12	9	195
roasted	1	12	8	182
stewed	1	11	8	187
neck, meat & skin				
fried				
batter-dipped	1	16	12	172
flour-coated	1	11	9	119
simmered	1	10	7	94
neck, meat only				
fried	1	9	3	50
simmered	1	8	1	32
thigh, meat & skin				
fried				
batter-dipped	1	16	14	238
flour-coated	1	8	9	162
roasted	1	8	10	153
stewed	1	8	10	158

	Portion	Calcium (mg)	Total Fat (g)	Total Calor
thigh, meat only				
fried	1	7	5	113
roasted	1	6	6	109
stewed	1	6	5	107
wing, meat & skin				
fried				
batter-dipped	1	10	11	159
flour-coated	1	5	7	103
roasted	1	5	7	99
stewed	1	5	7	100
wing, meat only				
fried	1	3	2	42
roasted	1	3	2	43
stewed	1	3	2	43
CHICKEN, ROASTING				
flesh & skin, roasted	½ chicken	58	64	1,071
flesh only, roasted	1 c	16	9	233
giblets, simmered	1 c	18	7	239
light meat w/out skin, roasted	1 c	18	6	214
dark meat w/out skin, roasted	1 c	15	12	250
CHICKEN, STEWING				
flesh, skin, giblets, & neck, stewed	1 chicken	78	107	1,636
flesh & skin, stewed	½ chicken	33	49	744
flesh only, stewed	1 c	18	17	332
giblets, simmered	1 c	19	13	281
light meat w/out skin, stewed	1 c	19	11	298
dark meat w/out skin, stewed	1 c	17	21	361
CHICKEN, CAPONS				
flesh, skin, giblets, & neck, roasted	1 chicken	211	165	3,211
flesh & skin, roasted	½ chicken	91	74	1,457
giblets, simmered	1 c	19	8	238

Duck, Fresh

	Portion	Calcium (mg)	Total Fat (g)	Total Calor
DOMESTICATED				
flesh & skin, roasted	½ duck	43	108	1,287
flesh only, roasted	½ duck	26	25	445
WILD				
flesh & skin, raw	1 lb of ready-to-cook bird	11	36	505
breast, meat only, raw	½ breast	3	4	102

	Portion	Calcium (mg)	Total Fat (g)	Total Calor

Goose, Fresh, Domesticated

	Portion	Calcium (mg)	Total Fat (g)	Total Calor
flesh & skin, roasted	½ goose	104	170	2,362
flesh only, roasted	½ goose	84	75	1,406
liver, raw	1	40	4	125

Guinea, Fresh

	Portion	Calcium (mg)	Total Fat (g)	Total Calor
flesh & skin, raw	1 lb of ready-to-cook bird	?	23	568
flesh only, raw	1 lb of ready-to-cook bird	?	7	304

Pheasant, Fresh

	Portion	Calcium (mg)	Total Fat (g)	Total Calor
flesh & skin, raw	1 lb of ready-to-cook bird	46	34	670
flesh only, raw	1 lb of ready-to-cook bird	42	12	435
breast, meat only, raw	½ breast	6	6	243
leg, meat only, raw	1	31	5	143

Quail, Fresh

	Portion	Calcium (mg)	Total Fat (g)	Total Calor
flesh & skin, raw	1 quail	14	13	210
flesh only, raw	1 quail	12	4	123
breast, meat only, raw	1	5	2	69

Squab (Pigeon), Fresh

	Portion	Calcium (mg)	Total Fat (g)	Total Calor
flesh only, raw	1 squab	?	13	239
breast, meat only, raw	1	?	5	135

Turkey, Fresh

TURKEY, ALL CLASSES

	Portion	Calcium (mg)	Total Fat (g)	Total Calor
flesh, skin, giblets, & neck, roasted	1 lb of ready-to-cook bird	68	25	533
	1 turkey	1,049	380	8,245
flesh & skin, roasted	1 lb of ready-to-cook bird	63	23	498
	½ turkey	488	180	3,857
flesh only, roasted	1 c	35	7	238
skin only, roasted	½ turkey	87	98	1,096
giblets, simmered	1 c	18	7	243
gizzard, simmered	1 c	22	6	236
heart, simmered	1 c	19	9	257
liver, simmered	1 c	15	8	237
light meat w/skin, roasted	½ turkey	225	87	2,069
dark meat w/skin, roasted	½ turkey	263	93	1,789

	Portion	Calcium (mg)	Total Fat (g)	Total Calor
light meat w/out skin, roasted	1 c	27	5	219
dark meat w/out skin, roasted	1 c	45	10	262
back, meat & skin, roasted	½ back	87	38	637
breast, meat & skin, roasted	½ breast	182	64	1,637
leg, meat & skin, roasted	1	176	54	1,133
neck, meat only, simmered	1	56	11	274
wing, meat & skin, roasted	1	44	23	426

TURKEY, FRYER ROASTERS

	Portion	Calcium (mg)	Total Fat (g)	Total Calor
flesh, skin, giblets, & neck, roasted	1 lb of ready-to-cook bird	58	14	429
	1 turkey	409	100	3,029
flesh & skin, roasted	1 lb of ready-to-cook bird	51	13	395
	½ turkey	180	46	1,392
flesh only, roasted	1 lb of ready-to-cook bird	39	5	292
	1 c	28	4	210
skin only, roasted	½ turkey	43	28	362
light meat w/skin, roasted	½ turkey	77	20	711
dark meat w/skin, roasted	½ turkey	103	26	680
light meat w/out skin, roasted	1 c	20	2	195
dark meat w/out skin, roasted	1 c	37	6	227
back				
meat & skin, roasted	½ back	47	11	265
meat only, roasted	½ back	35	5	164
breast				
meat & skin, roasted	½ breast	51	11	526
meat only, roasted	½ breast	38	2	413
leg				
meat & skin, roasted	1	56	13	418
meat only, roasted	1	49	8	355
wing				
meat & skin, roasted	1	26	9	186
meat only, roasted	1	15	2	98

TURKEY, YOUNG HENS

	Portion	Calcium (mg)	Total Fat (g)	Total Calor
flesh, skin, giblets, & neck, roasted	1 lb of ready-to-cook bird	69	28	565
	1 turkey	860	348	7,094
flesh & skin, roasted	½ turkey	399	166	3,323
flesh only, roasted	1 c	35	8	244
skin only, roasted	½ turkey	64	87	945
light meat w/skin, roasted	½ turkey	195	81	1,778
dark meat w/skin, roasted	½ turkey	204	85	1,544
light meat w/out skin, roasted	1 c	29	5	226
dark meat w/out skin, roasted	1 c	42	11	268
back, meat & skin, roasted	½ back	67	34	551
breast, meat & skin, roasted	½ breast	152	54	1,330

	Portion	Calcium (mg)	Total Fat (g)	Total Calor
leg, meat & skin, roasted	1	136	47	955
wing, meat & skin, roasted	1	41	23	414
TURKEY, YOUNG TOMS				
flesh, skin, giblets & neck, roasted	1 lb of ready-to-cook bird	68	23	514
	1 turkey	1,578	525	11,873
flesh & skin, roasted	1 lb of ready-to-cook bird	64	22	482
	½ turkey	735	249	5,545
flesh only, roasted	1 c	35	7	235
skin only, roasted	½ turkey	139	139	1,578
light meat w/skin, roasted	½ turkey	323	121	2,992
dark meat w/skin, roasted	½ turkey	413	128	2,553
light meat w/out skin, roasted	1 c	25	4	215
dark meat w/out skin, roasted	1 c	48	10	260
back, meat & skin				
raw	½ back	88	58	940
roasted	½ back	133	52	903
breast, meat & skin, roasted	½ breast	273	98	2,510
leg, meat & skin, roasted	1	280	78	1,660
wing, meat & skin, roasted	1	54	27	524

Poultry, Processed

MECHANICALLY DEBONED POULTRY

	Portion	Calcium (mg)	Total Fat (g)	Total Calor
from broiler backs & necks				
w/skin, raw	½ lb	312	56	616
w/out skin, raw	½ lb	280	35	450
from mature hens, raw	½ lb	423	45	551
from turkey breast & rib bones, w/ or w/out backs, raw	½ lb	329	36	455
TURKEY				
gravy & turkey, frozen	5 oz	20	4	95
patties, breaded, battered, fried	2¼ oz	9	12	181
	3⅓ oz	13	17	266
prebasted turkey				
breast, meat & skin, roasted	½ breast	75	30	1,087
thigh, meat & skin, roasted	1	25	27	494
roasts, boneless, frozen, seasoned, light & dark meat, roasted	0.43 lb	10	11	304
	1.72 lb	40	45	1,213
sticks, breaded, battered, fried	1 stick = 2¼ oz	9	11	178

	Portion	Calcium (mg)	Total Fat (g)	Total Calor

- **BRAND NAME**

Land O'Lakes
TURKEY PARTS

breast	3 oz	<20	1	100
drumsticks	3 oz	<20	5	120
hindquarters roast	3 oz	<20	8	140
thighs	3 oz	<20	10	150
wings	3 oz	<20	5	120

TURKEY PRODUCTS

breast fillets w/cheese	5 oz	150	16	300
patties	2¼ oz	40	11	170
sticks	2 oz	20	10	150

WHOLE TURKEY

butter-basted young turkey	3 oz	<20	8	140
self-basting (broth) young turkey	3 oz	<20	5	120
young turkey	3 oz	<20	7	130

Tyson
FULLY COOKED CHICKEN

Batter Gold	about 3½ oz	33	19	285
buttermilk	about 3½ oz	56	20	285
Delecta Delicious	about 3½ oz	31	19	305
Heat N Serve (oven ready)	about 3½ oz	14	17	270
Honey Stung	about 3½ oz	12	14	260
lightly breaded	about 3½ oz	13	14	255

POULTRY PRODUCTS

breast patties	3 oz	?	17	240
breast strips	about 3½ oz	8	13	270
chicken pattie	about 3½ oz	18	19	275
Chick'n Cheddar	3 oz	?	17	260
Heat N Serve	about 3½ oz	9	19	280
Sandwich Mate	about 3½ oz	13	20	315
School Lunch pattie	about 3½ oz	42	20	290
Swiss 'n Bacon	3 oz	?	20	280

READY-TO-COOK POULTRY

boneless breast	about 3½ oz	4	13	205
Cornish & split Cornish	about 3½ oz	11	14	240
IQF chicken & split broilers	about 3½ oz	11	15	245
prebreaded marinated chicken	about 3½ oz	20	17	285

□ **POULTRY SPREADS** *See* **PROCESSED MEAT & POULTRY PRODUCTS**

	Portion	Calcium (mg)	Total Fat (g)	Total Calor

❏ **PRESERVES** *See* FRUIT SPREADS

❏ **PROCESSED MEAT & POULTRY PRODUCTS: SAUSAGES, FRANKFURTERS, COLD CUTS, PÂTÉS, & SPREADS**
See also BEEF, FRESH & CURED; PORK, FRESH & CURED; POULTRY, FRESH & PROCESSED

	Portion	Calcium (mg)	Total Fat (g)	Total Calor
bacon & Canadian-style bacon *See* PORK, FRESH & CURED				
barbecue loaf, pork, beef	1 oz	15	3	49
beef sausage, smoked	1 oz	2	8	89
	1½ oz	4	12	134
beerwurst, beer salami				
beef	0.2 oz	1	2	19
	0.8 oz	2	7	75
pork	0.2 oz	0	1	14
	0.8 oz	2	4	55
berliner, pork, beef	1 oz	3	5	65
blood sausage	1 oz	?	10	107
bockwurst, raw (pork, veal)	2½ oz	?	18	200
	1 oz	?	8	87
bologna				
beef	0.8 oz	3	7	72
	1 oz	3	8	89
beef & pork	0.8 oz	3	7	73
	1 oz	3	8	89
pork	0.8 oz	3	5	57
	1 oz	3	6	70
turkey	1 oz	24	4	57
bratwurst, cooked, pork	3 oz	38	22	256
	1 oz	13	7	85
braunschweiger (a liver sausage), pork	0.6 oz	2	6	65
	1 oz	2	9	102
breakfast strips *See* BEEF, FRESH & CURED; PORK, FRESH & CURED				
brotwurst, pork, beef	2½ oz	34	19	226
	1 oz	14	8	92
cheesefurter, pork, beef	1½ oz	25	12	141
chicken, canned, boned, w/ broth	5 oz	20	11	234
chicken roll, light meat	2 oz	24	4	90
	6 oz	73	13	271
chicken spread, canned	1 T	16	2	25
	1 oz	35	3	55
chorizo, pork & beef	1 oz	?	11	?
corned beef, braised *See* BEEF, FRESH & CURED				

	Portion	Calcium (mg)	Total Fat (g)	Total Calor
corned beef, canned	1 oz	?	4	71
corned beef loaf, jellied	1 oz	3	2	46
dried beef	1 oz	2	1	47
Dutch brand loaf, pork, beef	1 oz	24	5	68
frankfurter				
beef	2 oz	7	17	184
	1.6 oz	6	13	145
beef & pork	2 oz	6	17	183
	1.6 oz	5	13	144
chicken	1.6 oz	43	9	116
	1 oz	27	6	73
turkey	1.6 oz	48	8	102
	1 oz	30	5	64
ham, boneless or canned *See* PORK, FRESH & CURED				
ham, chopped	1 oz	2	5	65
ham, chopped, canned	1 oz	2	5	68
ham, minced	1 oz	3	6	75
ham & cheese loaf or roll	1 oz	16	6	73
ham & cheese spread	1 T	33	3	37
	1 oz	62	5	69
ham salad spread	1 T	1	2	32
	1 oz	2	4	61
head cheese, pork	1 oz	4	4	60
honey loaf, pork, beef	1 oz	5	1	36
honey roll sausage, beef	1 oz	3	3	52
hot dog *See* frankfurter, *above*				
Italian sausage, pork				
raw	3.2 oz	16	29	315
	4 oz	20	35	391
cooked	2.3 oz	16	17	216
	2.9 oz	20	21	268
kielbasa, pork, beef	1 oz	12	8	88
knockwurst, pork, beef	2.4 oz	7	19	209
	1 oz	3	8	87
Lebanon bologna, beef	0.8 oz	3	3	52
	1 oz	4	4	64
liver cheese, pork	1.3 oz	3	10	115
	1 oz	2	7	86
liver sausage (liverwurst), pork	1 oz	7	8	93
luncheon meat				
beef, jellied	1 oz	3	1	31
beef, loaved	1 oz	3	7	87
beef, thin-sliced	1 oz	?	1	35
pork, beef	1 oz	3	9	100
pork, canned	1 oz	2	9	95
luncheon sausage, pork & beef	0.8 oz	3	5	60
	1 oz	4	6	74
mortadella, beef, pork	about ½ oz	3	4	47
	1 oz	5	7	88
olive loaf, pork	1 oz	31	5	67

	Portion	Calcium (mg)	Total Fat (g)	Total Calor
pastrami				
beef	1 oz	2	8	99
turkey	2 oz	5	4	80
	8 oz	20	14	320
pâté				
chicken liver, canned	1 T	1	2	26
	1 oz	3	4	57
goose liver, smoked, canned	1 T	?	6	60
	1 oz	?	12	131
liver (not specified), canned	1 T	9	4	41
	1 oz	20	8	90
peppered loaf, pork, beef	1 oz	15	2	42
pepperoni, pork, beef	8.8 oz	25	110	1,248
	0.2 oz	1	2	27
pickle & pimento loaf, pork	1 oz	27	6	74
picnic loaf, pork, beef	1 oz	13	5	66
Polish sausage, pork	8 oz	26	65	739
	1 oz	3	8	92
pork & beef sausage, fresh,	about 1 oz	?	10	107
cooked	about ½ oz	?	5	52
pork sausage, country style,	about 1 oz	9	8	100
fresh, cooked	about ½ oz	4	4	48
salami				
cooked				
beef	0.8 oz	2	5	58
	1 oz	2	6	72
beef & pork	0.8 oz	3	5	57
	1 oz	4	6	71
turkey	2 oz	11	8	111
	8 oz	44	31	446
dry or hard				
pork	0.35 oz	1	3	41
	4 oz	15	38	460
pork, beef	0.35 oz	1	3	42
	4 oz	8	39	472
sandwich spread				
pork, beef	1 T	2	3	35
	1 oz	3	5	67
poultry salad	1 T	1	2	26
	1 oz	3	4	57
smoked chopped beef	1 oz	?	1	38
smoked link sausage				
pork, grilled	2.4 oz	20	22	265
	about ½ oz	5	5	62
pork & beef	2.4 oz	7	21	229
	about ½ oz	2	5	54
flour & nonfat dry milk	2.4 oz	12	15	182
added	about ½ oz	3	3	43
nonfat dry milk added	2.4 oz	28	19	213
	about ½ oz	6	4	50

	Portion	Calcium (mg)	Total Fat (g)	Total Calor
Thuringer, cervelat, summer	0.8 oz	2	7	80
sausage: beef, pork	1 oz	2	8	98
turkey				
canned, boned, w/broth	5 oz	17	10	231
diced, light & dark, seasoned	1 oz	0	2	39
	½ lb	2	14	313
turkey breast meat	0.7 oz	1	tr	23
turkey ham (cured turkey	2 oz	5	3	73
thigh meat)	8 oz	22	12	291
turkey loaf, breast meat	1½ oz	3	1	47
	6 oz	12	3	187
turkey pastrami See pastrami: turkey, above				
turkey roll, light meat	1 oz	11	2	42
turkey roll, light & dark meat	1 oz	9	2	42
Vienna sausage, canned, beef & pork	0.6 oz	2	4	45

• BRAND NAME

Carl Buddig Luncheon Meats
beef, chicken, turkey	1 oz	≤4	2–3	40–50
ham	1 oz	11	3	50

Land O'Lakes
diced turkey, white & dark mixed	3 oz	20	6	120
turkey ham	3 oz	<20	2	100

Louis Rich
barbecued breast of turkey	1 oz	2	1	38
hickory smoked breast of turkey	1 oz	1	1	35
oven roasted breast of turkey	1 oz	2	1	36
oven roasted chicken breast	1 oz	10	2	39
smoked turkey breast, sliced	¾ oz	1	tr	21
turkey franks	1 link = 1.58 oz	61	9	103
turkey ham	1 oz	2	1	34
turkey pastrami	1 oz	2	1	33
turkey salami	1 oz	6	4	52
turkey smoked sausage	1 oz	5	4	55

Oscar Mayer
FRANKFURTERS
beef	1 link	6	13	144
cheese	1 link	28	13	145
little wieners	1 link	1	3	28
wieners	1 link	5	13	144

	Portion	Calcium (mg)	Total Fat (g)	Total Calor
LUNCHEON MEATS				
Bar-B-Q loaf	1 oz	16	3	47
beef bologna	1 oz	3	8	90
beef cotto salami	0.8 oz	2	3	45
beef salami for beer	0.8 oz	2	6	67
beef summer sausage	0.8 oz	2	6	73
bologna	1 oz	3	8	90
braunschweiger liver sausage	1 oz	2	9	96
corned beef	0.6 oz	1	tr	16
cotto salami	0.8 oz	1	4	54
Genoa salami	0.3 oz	2	3	35
German brand braun-schweiger	1 oz	3	8	94
ham *See* PORK, FRESH & CURED				
ham & cheese loaf	1 oz	17	6	76
hard salami	0.3 oz	1	3	34
head cheese	1 oz	4	4	55
honey loaf	1 oz	6	1	35
Italian-style beef	0.6 oz	2	1	18
liver cheese	1.3 oz	3	10	116
luncheon meat	1 oz	3	9	99
Luxury Loaf	1 oz	11	1	38
New England brand sausage	0.8 oz	1	2	31
Old Fashioned Loaf	1 oz	28	4	64
olive loaf	1 oz	31	4	63
pastrami	0.6 oz	1	tr	17
peppered loaf	1 oz	13	2	43
pickle & pimiento loaf	1 oz	35	4	64
picnic loaf	1 oz	12	4	62
summer sausage	0.8 oz	2	7	73
SAUSAGES				
all	1 link	<6	varies	varies
SLICED CHICKEN & TURKEY				
smoked chicken breast	1 oz	2	1	27
smoked turkey breast	0.7 oz	2	tr	20
SPREADS				
braunschweiger liver sausage	1 oz	2	9	95
ham & cheese	1 oz	51	5	66
ham salad	1 oz	2	4	62
sandwich	1 oz	3	5	67
Swanson				
chunk premium white chicken, canned	2½ oz	<20	2	90
chunk-style Mixin' Chicken, canned	2½ oz	20	8	130

	Portion	Calcium (mg)	Total Fat (g)	Total Calor
chunk white & dark chicken, canned	2½ oz	<20	4	100
chunky chicken spread	1 oz	40	4	60
Tyson				
all white cooked chicken fryer meat	about 3½ oz	11	3	166
breast of chicken roll, whole & diced	about 3½ oz	6	9	155
chicken bologna	about 3½ oz	49	18	230
chicken corn dogs	about 3½ oz	49	14	280
chicken franks	about 3½ oz	35	25	285
Liberty Roll, whole & diced	about 3½ oz	10	12	185
natural proportioned cooked chicken meat	about 3½ oz	12	5	170

❑ **PUDDING DESSERTS, FROZEN**
See DESSERTS, FROZEN

❑ **PUDDINGS & PIE FILLINGS**
See DESSERTS: CUSTARDS, GELATINS,
PUDDINGS, & PIE FILLINGS

❑ **RELISHES** *See* PICKLES, OLIVES,
RELISHES, & CHUTNEYS

❑ **RICE & GRAINS, PLAIN & PREPARED**
See also VEGETABLES, PLAIN & PREPARED

barley, pearled, light, un-cooked	1 c	29	2	700
bulgur, uncooked	1 c	49	3	600
hominy grits *See* corn grits, *under* BREAKFAST CEREALS, COLD & HOT				
popcorn *See* SNACKS				
rice				
brown, cooked, hot	1 c	23	1	230
white, enriched				
raw	1 c	44	1	670
cooked, hot	1 c	21	tr	225
instant, ready-to-serve, hot	1 c	5	0	180
parboiled, raw	1 c	111	1	685
parboiled, cooked, hot	1 c	33	tr	185

	Portion	Calcium (mg)	Total Fat (g)	Total Calor
• BRAND NAME				
Arrowhead Mills				
PLAIN RICE & GRAINS				
barley, pearled	2 oz	<20	1	200
barley flakes	2 oz	<20	1	200
buckwheat groats				
brown	2 oz	60	1	190
white	2 oz	<20	1	190
bulgur wheat	2 oz	20	1	200
millet	2 oz	<20	1	90
oat flakes	2 oz	20	4	220
oat groats	2 oz	40	4	220
quinoa	2 oz	60	3	200
rice, brown: long, long basmati, medium, or short	2 oz	20	1	200
rye or rye flakes	2 oz	20	1	190
triticale or triticale flakes	2 oz	20	1	190
wheat, hard, red, winter, or soft pastry	2 oz	20	1	190
wheat flakes	2 oz	40	1	210
PREPARED RICE & GRAINS				
quick brown rice				
regular	2 oz	20	1	200
Spanish style	¼ of 5.65 oz pkg	20	1	150
vegetable herb	¼ of 5.6 oz pkg	20	1	150
wild rice & herbs	¼ of 5.35 oz pkg	20	1	140
Birds Eye International Rice Recipes				
French style	3.3 oz	<20	0	110
Italian style	3.3 oz	<20	1	120
Spanish style	3.3 oz	<20	0	110
Carolina Rice				
extra long grain, enriched	about ½ c cooked	<20	0	100
long grain, enriched, precooked instant	about ½ c cooked	<20	0	110
Chun King				
rice mix	¼ oz	<20	0	20
Fearn				
Naturfresh corn germ	¼ c or 1 oz	<20	7	130
Naturfresh raw wheat germ	¼ c or 1 oz	20	3	100
Health Valley				
amaranth pilaf, regular or low salt	4 oz	20	3	90

	Portion	Calcium (mg)	Total Fat (g)	Total Calor
Mahatma				
long grain rice, enriched	about ½ c cooked	<20	0	100
long grain rice, enriched, pre-cooked instant	about ½ c cooked	<20	0	110
natural long grain rice, brown	about ½ c cooked	<20	0	110
Minute Rice				
all rice & mixes	½ c	<20	4–5	120–160
Pillsbury Frozen Rice Originals				
Italian blend white rice & spinach in cheese sauce	½ c	60	7	170
long grain white & wild rice	½ c	0	2	120
Rice Jubilee	½ c	0	6	150
Rice Medley	½ c	0	3	120
rice & broccoli in flavored cheese sauce	½ c	40	4	120
rice pilaf	½ c	0	2	120
rice w/herb butter sauce	½ c	0	5	150
Quaker Oats				
Scotch brand medium or quick pearled barley	¼ c	11	1	172
Rice-A-Roni				
MICROWAVE LONG GRAIN & WILD RICE MIXES				
original flavor w/herbs & seasoning, prepared	½ c	<20	4	140
chicken flavor & mushroom, prepared	½ c	<20	4	140
RICE & PASTA MIXES				
beef flavor, prepared	½ c	<20	5	170
beef flavor & mushroom, prepared	½ c	<20	4	150
chicken & mushroom flavor, prepared	½ c	<20	7	180
chicken flavor, prepared	½ c	<20	5	170
chicken flavor/chicken broth w/herbs, twin pack, prepared	⅔ c	<20	7	220
chicken flavor & vegetables, prepared	½ c	<20	4	140
fried rice w/almonds, prepared	½ c	<20	5	140
herbs & butter, prepared	½ c	20	4	130
rice pilaf, prepared	½ c	20	6	190
risotto, prepared	¾ c	<20	7	210
Spanish rice, prepared	½ c	<20	4	140

	Portion	Calcium (mg)	Total Fat (g)	Total Calor
Stroganoff w/sour cream sauce, prepared	½ c	20	8	200
RICE MIXES				
brown & wild rice w/mushrooms, prepared	½ c	<20	8	180
long grain & wild rice w/ herbs & seasoning, prepared	½ c	20	5	140
yellow rice dinner, prepared	¾ c	<20	7	250
River				
enriched rice	about ½ c cooked	<20	0	100
natural long grain rice, brown	about ½ c cooked	<20	0	110
Riviana Make-It-Easy				
beef-flavored rice & vermicelli mix	⅛ of 8 oz box or about ½ c cooked	<20	1	130
chicken-flavored rice & vermicelli mix	⅛ of 8 oz box or about ½ c cooked	<20	1	130
Stouffer				
apple pecan rice	½ of 5⅞ oz pkg	<20	4	130
Rice Medley	3 oz	<20	2	110
Success				
enriched, precooked, natural long grain rice	about ½ c cooked	<20	0	100
Van Camp's				
Golden Hominy	1 c	9	1	128
Spanish rice	1 c	35	3	150
Water Maid				
enriched rice	about ½ c cooked	<20	0	100

❏ **ROLLS** *See* BREADS, ROLLS, BISCUITS, & MUFFINS

❏ **SALAD DRESSINGS, MAYONNAISE, VINEGAR, & DIPS**

Mayonnaise, Commercial

mayonnaise				
safflower & soybean	1 c	40	175	1,577
	1 T	2	11	99

	Portion	Calcium (mg)	Total Fat (g)	Total Calor
soybean	1 c	40	175	1,577
	1 T	2	11	99
mayonnaise-type dressing				
regular	1 c	33	78	916
	1 T	2	5	57
low-cal	1 T	3	2	19

Salad Dressings

	Portion	Calcium (mg)	Total Fat (g)	Total Calor
bleu cheese, commercial				
regular	1 c	199	128	1,235
	1 T	12	8	77
low-cal	1 T	9	1	11
cooked, homemade	1 c	214	24	400
	1 T	13	2	25
French				
commercial				
regular	1 c	28	102	1,074
	1 T	2	6	67
creamy	1 T	1	7	70
low-cal	1 c	29	15	349
	1 T	2	1	22
homemade	1 c	13	154	1,388
	1 T	1	10	88
Green Goddess, commercial	1 T	2	7	68
Italian, commercial				
regular	1 c	23	114	1,098
	1 T	1	7	69
creamy	1 T	0	5	52
low-cal	1 c	5	24	253
	1 T	0	2	16
Russian, commercial				
regular	1 c	47	125	1,210
	1 T	3	8	76
low-cal	1 c	49	10	368
	1 T	3	1	23
sweet & sour, commercial	1 T	1	tr	29
Thousand Island, commercial				
regular	1 c	28	89	943
	1 T	2	6	59
low-cal	1 c	27	26	389
	1 T	2	2	24

Vinegar

	Portion	Calcium (mg)	Total Fat (g)	Total Calor
cider	1 T	1	0	tr
distilled	1 T	?	0	2

	Portion	Calcium (mg)	Total Fat (g)	Total Calor

• BRAND NAME

Good Seasons Salad Dressing Mixes

	Portion	Calcium (mg)	Total Fat (g)	Total Calor
bleu cheese & herbs, w/vinegar, water, & salad oil	1 T	<20	9	80
Buttermilk Farm Style, w/ whole milk & mayonnaise	1 T	<20	6	60
cheese garlic, w/vinegar, water, & salad oil	1 T	<20	9	80
cheese Italian, w/vinegar, water, & salad oil	1 T	<20	9	80
classic herb, w/vinegar, water, & salad oil	1 T	<20	9	80
garlic & herbs, w/vinegar, water, & salad oil	1 T	<20	9	80
Italian, w/vinegar, water, & salad oil	1 T	<20	9	80
lemon & herbs, w/vinegar, water, & salad oil	1 T	<20	9	80
lite Italian, w/vinegar, water, & salad oil	1 T	<20	3	25
no-oil Italian, w/vinegar & water	1 T	<20	0	6

Hellman's

	Portion	Calcium (mg)	Total Fat (g)	Total Calor
Real mayonnaise	1 T	<20	11	100
sandwich spread	1 T	<20	5	50
tartar sauce	1 T	<20	8	70

Land O'Lakes

	Portion	Calcium (mg)	Total Fat (g)	Total Calor
dips, flavored, dairy	2 oz	60	5	70

Life All Natural

	Portion	Calcium (mg)	Total Fat (g)	Total Calor
avocado dressing/dip w/tofu	½ oz	<20	7	70
creamy salad dressing, egg-free, low-cholesterol	½ oz	<20	4	39
garlic dressing/dip w/tofu	½ oz	<20	7	70
mayonnaise-style dressing, egg-free, low-cholesterol	½ oz	<20	8	71
tofu dressing/dip	½ oz	<20	7	75

Ortega

	Portion	Calcium (mg)	Total Fat (g)	Total Calor
Acapulco Dip	1 oz	<20	0	8

Regina

	Portion	Calcium (mg)	Total Fat (g)	Total Calor
wine vinegars, all flavors	1 fl oz	<20	0	4

❑ SALADS, COMMERCIALLY PREPARED
See FAST FOODS; FRUIT, FRESH
& PROCESSED; VEGETABLES, PLAIN
& PREPARED

	Portion	Calcium (mg)	Total Fat (g)	Total Calor

❏ **SAUCES, DESSERT** *See* DESSERT
SAUCES, SYRUPS, & TOPPINGS

❏ **SAUCES, GRAVIES, & CONDIMENTS**
See also FRUIT, FRESH & PROCESSED; PICKLES,
OLIVES, RELISHES, & CHUTNEYS

Condiments

catsup	1 c	60	1	290
mustard, prepared, yellow	1 t	4	tr	5

Gravies

au jus				
canned	1 c	10	tr	38
	10½ oz	12	1	48
dehydrated, prepared w/ water	1 c	11	1	19
	21.7 oz	27	2	48
beef, canned	1 c	14	5	124
	10¼ oz	17	7	155
brown, dehydrated, prepared w/water	1 c	7	tr	9
	9.7 oz	8	tr	9
chicken				
canned	1 c	48	14	189
	10½ oz	60	17	236
dehydrated, prepared w/ water	1 c	39	2	83
mushroom				
canned	1 c	17	6	120
	10½ oz	22	8	150
dehydrated, prepared w/ water	1 c	49	1	70
onion, dehydrated, prepared w/water	1 c	69	1	80
pork, dehydrated, prepared w/water	1 c	32	2	76
turkey				
canned	1 c	10	5	122
	10½ oz	12	6	152
dehydrated, prepared w/ water	1 c	50	2	87

	Portion	Calcium (mg)	Total Fat (g)	Total Calor
Sauces				
barbecue, ready-to-serve	1 c	48	5	188
béarnaise				
dehydrated	0.9 oz	?	2	90
dehydrated, prepared w/milk	1 c	?	68	701
& butter	13½ oz	?	102	1,052
cheese				
dehydrated	1.2 oz	280	9	158
dehydrated, prepared w/	1 c	570	17	307
whole milk				
curry				
dehydrated	1.2 oz	?	8	151
dehydrated, prepared w/	1 c	485	15	270
whole milk	12 oz	606	18	337
hollandaise, dehydrated				
w/butterfat	1.2 oz	97	16	187
w/butterfat, prepared w/	1 c	124	20	237
water	7.2 oz	97	16	187
w/vegetable oil	1 oz	?	2	93
w/vegetable oil, prepared w/	1 c	?	68	703
milk & butter	13½ oz	?	102	1,055
marinara, canned	1 c	44	8	171
	15½ oz	78	15	300
mushroom				
dehydrated	1 oz	?	3	99
dehydrated, prepared w/	1 c	?	10	228
whole milk	11.7 oz	?	13	285
sour cream				
dehydrated	1.2 oz	128	11	180
dehydrated, prepared w/	1 c	546	30	509
whole milk	5½ oz	273	15	255
soy *See* SOYBEANS & SOYBEAN PRODUCTS				
spaghetti				
canned	1 c	70	12	272
	15½ oz	124	21	479
dehydrated	0.35 oz	17	tr	28
	1½ oz	72	tr	118
dehydrated, w/mushrooms	0.35 oz	40	1	30
	1.4 oz	156	4	118
Stroganoff				
dehydrated	1.6 oz	307	4	161
dehydrated, prepared w/	1 c	521	11	271
whole milk & water	11.2 oz	562	12	292
sweet & sour				
dehydrated	2 oz	30	tr	220
dehydrated, prepared w/	1 c	41	tr	294
water & vinegar	8.3 oz	30	tr	220

	Portion	Calcium (mg)	Total Fat (g)	Total Calor
tamari *See* SOYBEANS & SOYBEAN PRODUCTS				
teriyaki *See* SOYBEANS & SOYBEAN PRODUCTS				
tomato, canned	½ c	17	tr	37
Spanish style	½ c	20	tr	40
w/herbs & cheese	½ c	45	2	72
w/mushrooms	½ c	16	tr	42
w/onions	½ c	20	tr	52
w/onions, green peppers, & celery	½ c	16	1	50
w/tomato tidbits	½ c	13	tr	39
tomato paste & puree *See* VEGETABLES, PLAIN & PREPARED				
white				
dehydrated	1.7 oz	334	13	230
dehydrated, prepared w/ whole milk	1 c	424	13	241
	23.2 oz	1,060	34	602

▪ BRAND NAME

A-1

steak sauce	1 T	<20	0	12

Chun King

mustard, brown	1 t	<20	0	4
sauce/glaze mix for sweet & sour entree	3.8 oz	100	0	370
sweet & sour sauce	1.8 oz	<20	0	60

Escoffier

Sauce Diable	1 T	<20	0	20
Sauce Robert	1 T	<20	0	20

Franco-American Gravies

au jus	2 oz	20	0	5
beef	2 oz	<20	1	25
brown, w/onions	2 oz	<20	1	25
chicken	2 oz	<20	4	50
chicken giblet	2 oz	<20	2	30
mushroom	2 oz	<20	1	25
pork	2 oz	<20	3	40
turkey	2 oz	<20	2	30

Fresh Chef Sauces

Bolognese	4 oz	40	7	130
pesto	4 oz	350	60	630
red clam	4 oz	20	4	90
tomato	4 oz	60	11	160
white clam	4 oz	20	10	130

Grey Poupon

Dijon mustard	1 T	<20	1	18

	Portion	Calcium (mg)	Total Fat (g)	Total Calor
Health Valley				
Catch-Up, regular or no salt	1 T	3	tr	16
tomato sauce, regular or no salt	4 oz	25	0	30
Life All Natural				
English mustard	¼ oz	<20	1	11
horseradish sauce	¼ fl oz	<20	tr	7
steak sauce	½ oz	100	tr	11
tartar sauce, egg-free, low-cholesterol	¼ fl oz	<20	2	19
tomato catsup	½ oz	<20	0	11
Worcestershire sauce	¼ oz	<20	tr	5
Open Pit				
all barbecue sauces	1 T	<20	0	25
Ortega				
enchilada sauce, mild or hot	1 oz	<20	0	12
green chile salsa				
mild or medium	1 oz	<20	0	8
hot	1 oz	<20	0	10
Picante salsa	1 oz	<20	0	10
Ranchera salsa	1 oz	20	0	12
taco salsa, mild or hot	1 oz	<20	0	10
taco sauce, mild or hot	1 oz	<20	0	12
Western-style taco sauce	1 oz	<20	0	8
Prego				
Al Fresco Garden tomato sauce	4 oz	20	5	100
Prego Plus				
w/beef sirloin & onion	4 oz	40	7	160
w/mushrooms & chunk	4 oz	40	5	130
w/sausage & green peppers	4 oz	40	9	170
w/veal & sliced mushrooms	4 oz	40	5	150
spaghetti sauce	4 oz	20	6	140
spaghetti sauce, meat-flavored	4 oz	20	6	150
Steak Supreme				
steak sauce	1 T	<20	0	20
Tabasco				
Tabasco sauce	¼ t	tr	tr	1
Wolf				
chili hot dog sauce	about ⅙ c	16	2	44

❑ SEAFOOD & SEAFOOD PRODUCTS

See also DINNERS, FROZEN; ENTREES & MAIN
COURSES, FROZEN

	Portion	Calcium (mg)	Total Fat (g)	Total Calor

Finfish

ahi *See* tuna: yellowfin, *below*
aku *See* tuna: skipjack, *below*

anchovy, European

raw	3 oz	125	4	111
canned in oil, drained solids	5	46	2	42
bass, freshwater, mixed species, raw	3 oz	68	3	97
bluefish, raw	3 oz	6	4	105
burbot, raw	3 oz	43	1	76

carp

raw	3 oz	35	5	108
baked, broiled, microwaved	3 oz	44	6	138

catfish, channel

raw	3 oz	34	4	99
breaded & fried	3 oz	37	11	194

chub *See* cisco, smoked, *below*

cisco, smoked	1 oz	7	3	50
	3 oz	22	10	151

cod
 Atlantic

raw	3 oz	13	1	70
baked, broiled, microwaved	3 oz	12	1	89
canned, solids & liquids	3 oz	18	1	89
dried & salted	1 oz	45	1	81
	3 oz	136	2	246
Pacific, raw	3 oz	6	1	70

croaker, Atlantic

raw	3 oz	13	3	89
breaded & fried	3 oz	27	11	188
cusk, raw	3 oz	9	1	74

dogfish *See* shark, *below*

drum, freshwater, raw	3 oz	51	4	101

eel, mixed species

raw	3 oz	17	10	156
baked, broiled, microwaved	3 oz	22	13	200

flatfish

raw	3 oz	15	1	78
baked, broiled, microwaved	3 oz	16	1	99

flounder *See* flatfish, *above*

grouper, mixed species

raw	3 oz	23	1	78
baked, broiled, microwaved	3 oz	18	1	100

haddock

raw	3 oz	28	1	74
baked, broiled, microwaved	3 oz	36	1	95
smoked	1 oz	14	tr	33
	3 oz	41	1	99

hake *See* whiting, *below*

	Portion	Calcium (mg)	Total Fat (g)	Total Calor
halibut				
Atlantic or Pacific				
raw	3 oz	40	2	93
baked, broiled, microwaved	3 oz	51	2	119
Greenland, raw	3 oz	3	12	158
herring				
Atlantic				
raw	3 oz	49	8	134
baked, broiled, microwaved	3 oz	63	10	172
canned *See* sardine: Atlantic, *below*				
kippered	1.4 oz	33	5	87
pickled	½ oz	12	3	39
lake *See* cisco, *above*				
jack *See* mackerel: jack, *below*				
ling, raw	3 oz	29	1	74
lingcod, raw	3 oz	12	1	72
lox *See* salmon: chinook, smoked, *below*				
mackerel				
Atlantic				
raw	3 oz	10	12	174
baked, broiled, microwaved	3 oz	13	15	223
jack, canned, drained solids	1 c	458	12	296
king, raw	3 oz	26	2	89
Pacific & jack, mixed species, raw	3 oz	19	7	133
Spanish				
raw	3 oz	10	5	118
baked, broiled, microwaved	3 oz	11	5	134
milkfish, raw	3 oz	43	6	126
monkfish, raw	3 oz	7	1	64
mullet, striped				
raw	3 oz	34	3	99
baked, broiled, microwaved	3 oz	26	4	127
ocean perch, Atlantic				
raw	3 oz	91	1	80
baked, broiled, microwaved	3 oz	117	2	103
perch, mixed species				
raw	3 oz	68	1	77
baked, broiled, microwaved	3 oz	87	1	99
pike				
northern				
raw	3 oz	48	1	75
baked, broiled, microwaved	3 oz	62	1	96
walleye, raw	3 oz	94	1	79
pollock				
Atlantic, raw	3 oz	51	1	78
walleye				
raw	3 oz	4	1	68
baked, broiled, microwaved	3 oz	5	1	96
pompano, Florida				
raw	3 oz	19	8	140

	Portion	Calcium (mg)	Total Fat (g)	Total Calor
baked, broiled, microwaved	3 oz	36	10	179
porgy *See* scup, *below*				
pout, ocean, raw	3 oz	8	1	67
redfish *See* ocean perch, *above*				
rockfish, Pacific, mixed species				
raw	3 oz	8	1	80
baked, broiled, microwaved	3 oz	10	2	103
salmon				
Atlantic, raw	3 oz	10	5	121
chinook				
raw	3 oz	19	9	153
smoked	1 oz	3	1	33
	3 oz	9	4	99
chum				
raw	3 oz	9	3	102
canned, drained solids w/	3 oz	212	5	120
bone	13 oz	920	20	521
pink, canned, solids w/bone	3 oz	181	5	118
& liquid	16 oz	969	27	631
red *See* salmon: sockeye, *below*				
sockeye				
raw	3 oz	5	7	143
baked, broiled, microwaved	3 oz	6	9	183
canned, drained solids w/	3 oz	203	6	130
bone	13 oz	883	27	566
sardine				
Atlantic, canned in oil,	2 sardines =	92	3	50
drained solids w/bone	0.8 oz			
	3.2 oz	351	11	192
Pacific, canned in tomato	1 sardine =	91	5	68
sauce, drained solids w/	1.3 oz			
bone	13 oz	887	44	658
scrod *See* cod: Atlantic, *above*				
scup, raw	3 oz	34	2	89
sea bass, mixed species				
raw	3 oz	9	2	82
baked, broiled, microwaved	3 oz	11	2	105
sea trout, mixed species, raw	3 oz	15	3	88
shad, American, raw	3 oz	40	12	167
shark, mixed species				
raw	3 oz	29	4	111
batter-dipped & fried	3 oz	42	12	194
sheepshead				
raw	3 oz	18	2	92
baked, broiled, microwaved	3 oz	32	1	107
smelt, rainbow				
raw	3 oz	51	2	83
baked, broiled, microwaved	3 oz	65	3	106
snapper, mixed species				
raw	3 oz	27	1	85
baked, broiled, microwaved	3 oz	34	1	109

	Portion	Calcium (mg)	Total Fat (g)	Total Calor
sole *See* flatfish, *above*				
spot, raw	3 oz	12	4	105
sucker, white, raw	3 oz	60	2	79
sunfish, pumpkinseed, raw	3 oz	68	1	76
swordfish				
raw	3 oz	4	3	103
baked, broiled, microwaved	3 oz	5	4	132
tilefish				
raw	3 oz	22	2	81
baked, broiled, microwaved	3 oz	22	4	125
trout				
mixed species, raw	3 oz	36	6	126
rainbow				
raw	3 oz	57	3	100
baked, broiled, microwaved	3 oz	73	4	129
tuna				
light				
canned in soybean oil,	3 oz	11	7	169
drained solids	6 oz	23	14	339
canned in water, drained	3 oz	10	tr	111
solids	5.8 oz	20	1	216
skipjack, raw	3 oz	24	1	88
white, canned in soybean	3 oz	4	7	158
oil, drained solids	6.3 oz	8	14	331
yellowfin, raw	3 oz	14	1	92
turbot				
domestic *See* halibut: Greenland, *above*				
European, raw	3 oz	15	3	81
whitefish, mixed species,	1 oz	5	tr	30
smoked	3 oz	15	1	92
whiting, mixed species				
raw	3 oz	41	1	77
baked, broiled, microwaved	3 oz	53	1	98

Shellfish

	Portion	Calcium (mg)	Total Fat (g)	Total Calor
abalone, mixed species				
raw	3 oz	27	1	89
fried	3 oz	32	6	161
clams, mixed species				
raw	3 oz	39	1	63
	9 large (50/qt) or 20 small (110/qt)	83	2	133
boiled, poached, steamed	3 oz	78	2	126
	20 small (110/qt)	83	2	133
breaded & fried	3 oz	54	9	171
	20 small (110/qt)	119	21	379

	Portion	Calcium (mg)	Total Fat (g)	Total Calor
canned, drained solids	3 oz	78	2	126
	1 c	148	3	236
canned, liquid	3 oz	11	tr	2
	1 c	31	tr	6
crab				
Alaska king				
raw	3 oz	39	1	71
	1 leg = 1 lb	80	1	144
boiled, poached, steamed	3 oz	50	1	82
	1 leg = 1 lb	80	2	129
blue				
raw	1 crab = ⅓ lb	19	tr	18
	3 oz	76	1	74
boiled, poached, steamed	3 oz	88	2	87
	1 c not packed	140	2	138
canned, dry pack or drained solids of wet pack	3 oz	86	1	84
	1 c not packed	137	2	133
Dungeness, raw	3 oz	39	1	73
	1 crab = 1½ lb	75	2	140
queen, raw	3 oz	22	1	76
crayfish, mixed species				
raw	3 oz	20	1	76
boiled, poached, steamed	3 oz	26	1	97
cuttlefish, mixed species, raw	3 oz	77	1	67
lobster, northern: boiled,	3 oz	52	1	83
poached, steamed	1 c	88	1	142
mussels, blue				
raw	3 oz	22	2	73
	1 c	39	3	129
boiled, poached, steamed	3 oz	28	4	147
octopus, common, raw	3 oz	45	1	70
oysters				
eastern				
raw	6 medium (70/qt)	38	2	58
	1 c	111	6	170
boiled, poached, steamed	6 medium (70/qt)	38	2	58
	3 oz	76	4	117
breaded & fried	3 oz	53	11	167
	6 medium (70/qt)	54	11	173
canned, solids & liquids	3 oz	38	2	58
	1 c	111	6	170

	Portion	Calcium (mg)	Total Fat (g)	Total Calor
oysters *(cont.)*				
Pacific, raw	1 medium (20/qt)	4	1	41
	3 oz	7	2	69
scallops, mixed species				
raw	2 large (30/ lb) or 5 small (75/lb)	7	tr	26
	3 oz	21	1	75
breaded & fried	2 large (30/ lb)	13	3	67
shrimp, mixed species				
raw	4 large (32/ lb)	15	tr	30
	3 oz	44	1	90
boiled, poached, steamed	4 large (32/ lb)	9	tr	22
	3 oz	32	1	84
breaded & fried	4 large (32/ lb)	20	4	73
	3 oz	57	10	206
canned, dry pack or drained	3 oz	50	2	102
solids of wet pack	1 c	75	3	154
snail, sea *See* whelk, *below*				
spiny lobster, mixed species,	3 oz	41	1	95
raw	1 lobster = 2 lb	102	3	233
squid, mixed species				
raw	3 oz	27	1	78
fried	3 oz	33	6	149
whelk				
raw	3 oz	48	tr	117
boiled, poached, steamed	3 oz	96	1	233

Seafood Products

	Portion	Calcium (mg)	Total Fat (g)	Total Calor
crab cakes (blue crab)	2.1 oz	63	6	93
fish sticks (walleye pollock), frozen, reheated	1 stick = 1 oz	6	3	76
gefilte fish, commercial, sweet recipe w/broth	1½ oz	10	1	35
imitation seafood, made from surimi				
crab, Alaska king	3 oz	11	1	87
scallops, mixed species	3 oz	7	tr	84
shrimp, mixed species	3 oz	16	1	86
surimi (processed from walleye pollock)	1 oz	2	tr	28
	3 oz	7	1	84
tuna salad	3 oz	15	8	159
	1 c	35	19	383

	Portion	Calcium (mg)	Total Fat (g)	Total Calor
BRAND NAME				
Fresh Chef				
seafood pasta salad	4¼ oz	40	17	240
Health Valley				
Best of Sea Food tuna	6½ oz	30	3	180
No Salt Diet tuna	6½ oz	30	3	200
Rokeach				
Natural Broth gefilte fish	1 ball = 2 oz	32	1	46
Old Vienna gefilte fish	1 ball = 2.6 oz	28	2	68
Old Vienna whitefish & pike gefilte fish	1 ball = 2.6 oz	23	1	70
whitefish & pike gefilte fish in jellied broth	1 ball = 2 oz	32	1	46

❏ SEASONINGS

See also BREADCRUMBS, CROUTONS, STUFFINGS, &
SEASONED COATINGS; SAUCES, GRAVIES, & CONDIMENTS;
VEGETABLES, PLAIN & PREPARED

	Portion	Calcium (mg)	Total Fat (g)	Total Calor
allspice, ground	1 t	13	tr	5
anise seed	1 t	14	tr	7
basil, ground	1 t	30	tr	4
bay leaf, crumbled	1 t	5	tr	2
caraway seed	1 t	14	tr	7
cardamon, ground	1 t	8	tr	6
celery seed	1 t	35	1	8
chervil, dried	1 t	8	0	1
chili pepper	1 t	2	tr	9
chili powder	1 t	7	tr	8
cinnamon, ground	1 t	28	tr	6
cinnamon sugar	1 t	?	tr	16
cloves, ground	1 t	14	tr	7
coriander leaf, dried	1 t	7	tr	2
coriander seed	1 t	13	tr	5
cumin seed	1 t	20	1	8
curry powder	1 t	10	tr	6
dill seed	1 t	32	tr	6
dillweed, dried	1 t	18	tr	3
fennel seed	1 t	24	tr	7
fenugreek seed	1 t	6	tr	12
garlic powder	1 t	2	tr	9
ginger, ground	1 t	2	tr	6
mace, ground	1 t	4	1	8
marjoram, dried	1 t	12	?	2

	Portion	Calcium (mg)	Total Fat (g)	Total Calor
mustard powder	1 t	5	1	9
mustard seed, yellow	1 t	17	1	15
nutmeg, ground	1 t	4	1	12
onion powder	1 t	8	tr	7
oregano, ground	1 t	24	tr	5
paprika	1 t	4	tr	6
parsley, dried	1 t	19	tr	4
pepper, black	1 t	9	tr	5
pepper, red/cayenne	1 t	3	tr	6
pepper, seasoned	1 t	?	tr	10
pepper, white	1 t	6	tr	7
poppy seed	1 t	41	1	15
poultry seasoning	1 t	15	tr	5
pumpkin pie spice	1 t	12	tr	6
rosemary, dried	1 t	15	tr	4
saffron	1 t	1	tr	2
sage, ground	1 t	12	tr	2
salt	1 t	2	tr	0
savory, ground	1 t	30	1	4
tarragon, ground	1 t	18	tr	5
thyme, ground	1 t	26	tr	4
tumeric, ground	1 t	4	tr	8

• BRAND NAME

	Portion	Calcium (mg)	Total Fat (g)	Total Calor
Diamond Crystal				
salt substitute	1 pkt	?	?	3
French's				
imitation butter flavor salt	1 t	?	1	8
onion salt	1 t	?	?	6
seafood seasoning	1 t	?	?	2
seasoning salt	1 t	?	0	2
Health Valley				
all purpose	1 t	19	1	11
chicken	1 t	21	tr	8
fish	1 t	23	tr	11
steak/ham	1 t	18	tr	6
vegetable	1 t	18	tr	13
Kikkoman				
teriyaki baste & glaze	1 t	tr	tr	9
Lawry's				
onion salt	1 t	?	tr	7
seasoning salt	1 t	?	tr	3
McCormick's				
Season-All salt	1 t	3	tr	4

	Portion	Calcium (mg)	Total Fat (g)	Total Calor
Morton				
lite salt	1 t	3	0	0
salt substitute	1 t	30	0	0
Norcliff Thayer				
No Salt	1 pkt	?	0	0
Ortega				
mild taco meat seasoning	1 oz	40	1	90
Shake 'n Bake Seasoning Mixture				
all	¼ pouch	<20	1–4	70–80

❑ SEEDS & SEED-BASED BUTTERS, FLOURS, & MEALS

See also NUTS & NUT-BASED BUTTERS, FLOURS, MEALS, MILKS, PASTES, & POWDERS

alfalfa seeds, sprouted, raw	1 c	10	tr	10
breadfruit seeds				
raw	1 oz	10	2	54
boiled	1 oz	17	1	48
roasted	1 oz	24	1	59
breadnuttree seeds				
raw	1 oz	28	tr	62
dried	1 oz	27	tr	104
chia seeds, dried	1 oz	150	7	134
cottonseed flour				
partially defatted	1 T	24	tr	18
	1 c	449	6	337
low-fat	1 oz	135	tr	94
cottonseed kernels, roasted	1 T	10	4	51
	1 c	149	54	754
cottonseed meal, partially defatted	1 oz	143	1	104
lotus seeds				
raw	1 oz	12	tr	25
dried	1 oz	46	1	94
	1 c	52	1	106
pumpkin & squash seeds				
whole, roasted	1 oz	16	6	127
	1 c	35	12	285
kernels				
dried	1 oz	12	13	154
	1 c	59	63	747
roasted	1 oz	12	12	148
	1 c	97	96	1,184

ramons *See* breadnuttree seeds, *above*

	Portion	Calcium (mg)	Total Fat (g)	Total Calor
safflower seed kernels, dried	1 oz	22	11	147
safflower seed meal, partially defatted	1 oz	22	1	97
sesame butter				
paste	1 oz	273	14	169
	1 T	154	8	95
tahini				
from raw & stone-ground kernels	1 oz	119	14	162
	1 T	63	7	86
from roasted & toasted kernels	1 oz	121	15	169
	1 T	64	8	89
from unroasted kernels	1 oz	40	16	173
	1 T	20	8	85
sesame flour				
high-fat	1 oz	45	11	149
partially defatted	1 oz	43	3	109
low-fat	1 oz	42	1	95
sesame meal, partially defatted	1 oz	43	14	161
sesame seeds				
whole				
dried	1 T	88	4	52
	1 c	1,404	72	825
roasted & toasted	1 oz	281	14	161
kernels				
dried	1 T	10	4	47
	1 c	197	82	882
toasted	1 oz	37	14	161
sisymbrium sp. seeds, whole,	1 oz	464	1	90
dried	1 c	1,208	3	235
squash seeds *See* pumpkin & squash seeds, *above*				
sunflower seed butter	1 T	19	8	93
sunflower seed flour, partially	1 T	6	tr	16
defatted	1 c	91	1	261
sunflower seed kernels				
dried	1 oz	33	14	162
	1 c	168	71	821
dry roasted	1 oz	20	14	165
	1 c	90	64	745
oil roasted	1 oz	16	16	175
	1 c	76	78	830
toasted	1 oz	16	16	176
	1 c	76	76	829
tahini *See* sesame butter: tahini, *above*				
watermelon seed kernels,	1 oz	15	13	158
dried	1 c	59	51	602

	Portion	Calcium (mg)	Total Fat (g)	Total Calor

- **BRAND NAME**

Arrowhead Mills

alfalfa seeds, sprouted	1 c	20	1	40
amaranth seeds	2 oz	100	3	200
flax seeds	1 oz	80	10	140
sesame seeds				
whole	1 oz	350	14	160
hulled	1 oz	40	14	160
sesame tahini, chemical-free	1 oz	40	17	170
sunflower seeds, hulled	1 oz	40	13	160
Planters				
sunflower seeds	1 oz	20	14	160

❑ SHERBETS *See* DESSERTS, FROZEN

❑ SHORTENINGS *See* FATS, OILS, & SHORTENINGS

❑ SNACKS
See also CRACKERS

cheese puffs	1 oz	17	10	159
cheese straws	4	64	7	109
corn chips	1 oz	35	9	155
popcorn				
air-popped	1 c	1	tr	30
popped in vegetable oil	1 c	3	3	55
sugar-syrup-coated	1 c	2	1	135
potato chips	10	5	7	105
made from dried potatoes	1 oz	6	13	164
potato sticks	1 oz	5	10	148
	½ c	3	6	94
pretzels				
stick	10	1	tr	10
twisted, Dutch	1	4	1	65
twisted, thin	10	16	2	240
tortilla chips	1 oz	30	7	139

- **BRAND NAME**

Arrowhead Mills

popcorn, unpopped	2 oz	<20	3	210

	Portion	Calcium (mg)	Total Fat (g)	Total Calor
Cornnuts				
Original or unsalted	1 oz	<20	4	120
barbecue or nacho cheese	1 oz	<20	4	110
Del Monte				
pineapple nuggets	0.9 oz	<20	0	90
Sierra trail mix	0.9 oz	<20	7	130
tropical fruit mix	0.9 oz	<20	1	90
yogurt raisins, plain or strawberry	0.9 oz	40	5	120
Health Valley				
CORN CHIPS				
corn chips				
regular	1 oz	6	11	160
no salt	1 oz	4	11	160
cheese corn chips				
regular	1 oz	18	11	160
no salt	1 oz	16	10	160
POTATO CHIPS				
Country Chips, regular or no salt	1 oz	7	11	160
Country Ripples, regular or no salt	1 oz	7	11	160
potato chips, regular or no salt	1 oz	7	11	160
potato chips, dip, regular or no salt	1 oz	7	11	160
SNACK PUFFS				
Cheddar Lites				
regular or no salt	17	4	2	40
w/green onion	17	?	1	40
TORTILLA CHIPS				
Buenitos				
regular	1 oz	6	8	150
no salt	1 oz	4	8	150
nacho cheese & chili	1 oz	14	8	150
Mister Salty Pretzels				
butter-flavored sticks	90	<20	1	110
Dutch	2	<20	1	110
Junior	29	<20	2	110
Mini Mix	23	<20	1	110
sticks	90	<20	1	110
Veri-Thin sticks	45	<20	1	110

	Portion	Calcium (mg)	Total Fat (g)	Total Calor
Nabisco				
DOO DADS				
Original	1 oz or ½ c	20	6	140
cheddar & herb	1 oz or ½ c	20	6	140
Zesty cheese	1 oz or ½ c	20	6	140
GREAT CRISPS!				
cheese & chive	9	<20	4	70
French onion	7	<20	4	70
Italian	9	20	4	70
nacho	8	<20	4	70
Real bacon	9	<20	4	70
savory garlic	8	20	3	70
sesame	9	20	4	70
sour cream & onion	8	20	4	70
tomato & celery	9	20	4	70
NIPS				
Real cheddar cheese	13	<20	3	70
pizza	20	<20	3	70
taco	14	<20	4	70
Pepperidge Farm				
SNACK STICKS				
Original	8	20	5	130
cheese	8	<20	6	130
sesame	8	<20	5	130
TINY GOLDFISH				
Original	45	<20	7	140
cheddar cheese	45	20	6	140
Planters				
Cheez Balls	1 oz	<20	11	160
Cheez Curls	1 oz	<20	11	160
corn chips	1 oz	40	10	160
Fruit 'n Nut Mix	1 oz	<20	9	150
popcorn	3 c popped	<20	0	20
microwave, butter	3 c popped	<20	10	140
microwave, natural	3 c popped	<20	9	140
Potato Crunchies	1¼ oz	<20	11	190
pretzels	1 oz	<20	1	110
round toast crackers	4	20	7	140
sour cream & onion puffs	1 oz	<20	10	160
square cheese crackers	4	20	7	140

❑ SOUPS, PREPARED

Canned

asparagus, cream of, condensed	1 can = 10¾ oz	70	10	210

	Portion	Calcium (mg)	Total Fat (g)	Total Calor
asparagus, cream of, condensed *(cont.)*				
prepared w/water	1 c	29	4	87
prepared w/whole milk	1 c	175	8	161
	1 can	424	20	392
bean, black, condensed	1 can = 11 oz	110	4	285
prepared w/water	1 c	45	2	116
bean w/bacon, condensed	1 can = 11½ oz	196	14	420
prepared w/water	1 c	81	6	173
bean w/frankfurter, condensed	1 can = 11¼ oz	210	17	454
prepared w/water	1 c	86	7	187
bean w/ham, chunky, ready-to-serve	1 c	79	9	231
	1 can = 19¼ oz	177	19	519
beef, chunky, ready-to-serve	1 c	31	5	171
	1 can = 19 oz	69	12	383
beef broth or bouillon, ready-to-serve	1 c	15	1	16
	1 can = 14 oz	25	1	27
beef mushroom, condensed	1 can = 10¾ oz	12	7	?
prepared w/water	1 c	5	3	?
beef noodle, condensed	1 can = 10¾ oz	36	7	204
prepared w/water	1 c	15	3	84
celery, cream of, condensed	1 can = 10¾ oz	98	14	219
prepared w/water	1 c	40	6	90
prepared w/whole milk	1 c	186	10	165
	1 can	451	24	400
cheese, condensed	1 can = 11 oz	345	25	377
prepared w/water	1 c	142	10	155
prepared w/whole milk	1 c	288	15	230
	1 can	698	35	558
chicken, chunky, ready-to-serve	1 c	24	7	178
	1 can = 10¾ oz	29	8	216
chicken, cream of, condensed	1 can = 10¾ oz	83	18	283
prepared w/water	1 c	34	7	116
prepared w/whole milk	1 c	180	11	191
	1 can	437	28	464
chicken & dumplings, condensed	1 can = 10½ oz	35	13	236
prepared w/water	1 c	15	6	97

	Portion	Calcium (mg)	Total Fat (g)	Total Calor
chicken broth, condensed	1 can = 10¾ oz	17	3	94
prepared w/water	1 c	9	1	39
chicken gumbo, condensed	1 can = 10¾ oz	59	3	137
prepared w/water	1 c	24	1	56
chicken mushroom, condensed	1 can = 10¾ oz	70	22	?
prepared w/water	1 c	29	9	?
chicken noodle				
chunky, ready-to-serve	1 c	24	6	?
	1 can = 19 oz	54	13	?
condensed	1 can = 10½ oz	32	6	182
prepared w/water	1 c	17	2	75
chicken noodle w/meatballs,	1 c	30	4	99
ready-to-serve	1 can = 20 oz	69	8	227
chicken rice				
chunky, ready-to-serve	1 c	35	3	127
	1 can = 19 oz	78	7	286
condensed	1 can = 10½ oz	42	5	146
prepared w/water	1 c	17	2	60
chicken vegetable				
chunky, ready-to-serve	1 c	25	5	167
	1 can = 19 oz	57	11	374
condensed	1 can = 10½ oz	43	7	181
prepared w/water	1 c	18	3	74
chili beef, condensed	1 can = 11¼ oz	105	16	411
prepared w/water	1 c	43	7	169
clam chowder (Manhattan)				
chunky, ready-to-serve	1 c	67	3	133
	1 can = 19 oz	151	8	299
condensed	1 can = 10¾ oz	56	5	187
prepared w/water	1 c	34	2	78
clam chowder (New England), condensed	1 can = 10¾ oz	99	6	214
prepared w/water	1 c	43	3	95
prepared w/whole milk	1 c	187	7	163
	1 can	453	16	396
consommé w/gelatin, condensed	1 can = 10½ oz	21	0	71
prepared w/water	1 c	8	0	29

	Portion	Calcium (mg)	Total Fat (g)	Total Calor
crab, ready-to-serve	1 c	65	2	76
	1 can = 13 oz.	99	2	114
escarole, ready-to-serve	1 c	32	2	27
	1 can = 19½ oz	72	4	61
gazpacho, ready-to-serve	1 c	24	2	57
	1 can = 13 oz	37	3	87
lentil w/ham, ready-to-serve	1 c	42	3	140
	1 can = 20 oz	96	6	320
minestrone				
chunky, ready-to-serve	1 c	61	3	127
	1 can = 19 oz	136	6	285
condensed	1 can = 10½ oz	83	6	202
prepared w/water	1 c	34	3	83
mushroom, cream of, condensed	1 can = 10¾ oz	78	23	313
prepared w/water	1 c	46	9	129
prepared w/whole milk	1 c	178	14	203
	1 can	432	33	494
mushroom barley, condensed	1 can = 10¾ oz	31	5	?
prepared w/water	1 c	13	2	?
mushroom w/beef stock, condensed	1 can = 10¾ oz	25	10	208
prepared w/water	1 c	10	4	85
onion, condensed	1 can = 10½ oz	64	4	138
prepared w/water	1 c	26	2	57
onion, cream of, condensed	1 can = 10¾ oz	82	13	?
prepared w/water	1 c	34	5	?
prepared w/whole milk	1 c	180	9	?
	1 can	436	23	?
oyster stew, condensed	1 can = 10½ oz	52	9	144
prepared w/water	1 c	22	4	59
prepared w/whole milk	1 c	167	8	134
	1 can	406	19	325
pea, green, condensed	1 can = 11¼ oz	66	7	398
prepared w/water	1 c	27	3	164
prepared w/whole milk	1 c	173	7	239
	1 can	420	17	579
pea, split, w/ham				
chunky, ready-to-serve	1 c	33	4	184
	1 can = 19 oz	74	9	413

	Portion	Calcium (mg)	Total Fat (g)	Total Calor
condensed	1 can = 11½ oz	53	11	459
prepared w/water	1 c	22	4	189
pepperpot, condensed	1 can = 10½ oz	57	11	251
prepared w/water	1 c	23	5	103
potato, cream of, condensed	1 can = 10¾ oz	48	6	178
prepared w/water	1 c	20	2	73
prepared w/whole milk	1 c	166	6	148
	1 can	402	16	360
Scotch broth, condensed	1 can = 10½ oz	37	6	195
prepared w/water	1 c	15	3	80
shrimp, cream of, condensed	1 can = 10¾ oz	43	13	219
prepared w/water	1 c	18	5	90
prepared w/whole milk	1 c	164	9	165
	1 can	397	23	400
stockpot, condensed	1 can = 11 oz	53	9	242
prepared w/water	1 c	22	4	100
tomato, condensed	1 can = 10¾ oz	32	5	208
prepared w/water	1 c	13	2	86
prepared w/whole milk	1 c	159	6	160
	1 can	386	15	389
tomato beef w/noodle, condensed	1 can = 10¾ oz	43	10	341
prepared w/water	1 c	18	4	140
tomato bisque, condensed	1 can = 11 oz	98	6	300
prepared w/water	1 c	40	3	123
prepared w/whole milk	1 c	186	7	198
	1 can	452	16	481
tomato rice, condensed	1 can = 11 oz	56	7	291
prepared w/water	1 c	23	3	120
turkey, chunky, ready-to-serve	1 c	50	4	136
	1 can = 18¾ oz	112	10	306
turkey noodle, condensed	1 can = 10¾ oz	28	5	168
prepared w/water	1 c	12	2	69
turkey vegetable, condensed	1 can = 10½ oz	40	7	179
prepared w/water	1 c	17	3	74

	Portion	Calcium (mg)	Total Fat (g)	Total Calor
vegetable, chunky, ready-to-serve	1 c	56	4	122
	1 can = 19 oz	126	8	274
vegetable, vegetarian, condensed	1 can = 10½ oz	52	5	176
prepared w/water	1 c	21	2	72
vegetable w/beef, condensed	1 can = 10¾ oz	41	5	192
prepared w/water	1 c	17	2	79
vegetable w/beef broth, condensed	1 can = 10½ oz	43	5	197
prepared w/water	1 c	18	2	81

Dehydrated

	Portion	Calcium (mg)	Total Fat (g)	Total Calor
asparagus, cream of, prepared w/water	1 c	?	2	59
	39.7 oz	?	8	265
bean w/bacon, prepared w/water	1 c	?	2	105
beef broth or bouillon				
cubed	1 cube = 0.1 oz	?	tr	6
prepared w/water	1 c	5	1	19
	6 fl oz	4	1	14
beef noodle, prepared w/water	1 c	5	1	41
	6 fl oz	4	1	30
cauliflower, prepared w/water	1 c	?	2	68
celery, cream of, prepared w/water	1 c	?	2	63
chicken, cream of, prepared w/water	1 c	76	5	107
	6 fl oz	57	4	80
chicken broth or bouillon				
cubed	1 cube = 0.2 oz	?	tr	9
prepared w/water	1 c	15	1	21
	6 fl oz	11	1	16
chicken noodle	1 pkt = 2.6 oz	154	6	257
	1 pkt = 0.4 oz	23	1	38
prepared w/water	1 c	32	1	53
chicken rice, prepared w/water	1 c	8	1	60
chicken vegetable, prepared w/water	1 c	?	1	49
	6 fl oz	?	1	37
clam chowder (Manhattan)	1 c	?	2	65
clam chowder (New England)	1 c	76	4	95
consommé, w/gelatin added, prepared w/water	1 c	?	tr	17
	39½ oz	?	tr	77
leek, prepared w/water	1 c	?	2	71
	36 fl oz	?	9	319

	Portion	Calcium (mg)	Total Fat (g)	Total Calor
minestrone, prepared w/water	1 c	?	2	79
	40.2 oz	?	8	358
mushroom	1 pkt regular = 2.6 oz	228	17	328
	1 pkt instant = 0.6 oz	51	4	74
prepared w/water	1 c	67	5	96
onion	1 pkt = 1.4 oz	55	2	115
	1 pkt = ¼ oz	10	tr	21
prepared w/water	1 c	13	1	28
oxtail, prepared w/water	1 c	?	3	71
	36 fl oz	?	11	318
pea, green or split	1 pkt = 4 oz	68	5	402
	1 pkt = 1 oz	17	1	100
prepared w/water	1 c	22	2	133
tomato (includes cream of tomato)	1 pkt = ¾ oz	40	2	77
prepared w/water	1 c	54	2	102
	6 fl oz	41	2	77
tomato vegetable (includes Italian vegetable & spring vegetable)	1 pkt = 1.4 oz	18	2	125
prepared w/water	1 c	8	1	55
	6 fl oz	6	1	41
vegetable, cream of, prepared w/water	1 c	?	6	105
	6 fl oz	?	4	79
vegetable beef, prepared w/water	1 c	?	1	53
	1 pkt = 40 oz	?	5	240

▪ BRAND NAME

Campbell
CHUNKY SOUPS, READY-TO-SERVE

	Portion	Calcium (mg)	Total Fat (g)	Total Calor
bean w/ham, Old Fashioned	11 oz	100	9	290
	9⅝ oz	80	8	260
beef	10¾ oz	20	5	190
	9½ oz	20	4	170
chicken, Old Fashioned	9½ oz	20	4	150
chicken mushroom, creamy	10½ oz	20	26	320
	9⅜ oz	20	24	280
chicken noodle	9½ oz	20	6	180
chicken noodle w/mushroom	10¾ oz	20	7	200
chicken rice	9½ oz	20	4	140
chicken vegetable	9½ oz	20	6	170
chili beef	11 oz	60	7	290
	9¾ oz	60	6	260

	Portion	Calcium (mg)	Total Fat (g)	Total Calor
clam chowder (Manhattan style)	10¾ oz	60	5	160
	9½ oz	40	4	150
clam chowder (New England style)	10¾ oz	40	17	290
	9½ oz	40	15	250
Fisherman chowder	10¾ oz	80	14	260
	9½ oz	60	13	230
minestrone	9½ oz	60	4	160
mushroom, creamy	10½ oz	20	22	260
	9⅜ oz	20	20	240
sirloin burger	10¾ oz	20	9	220
	9½ oz	20	8	200
split pea & ham	10¾ oz	20	6	230
	9½ oz	20	5	210
steak & potato	10¾ oz	<20	5	200
	9½ oz	<20	4	170
Stroganoff-style beef	10¾ oz	60	15	300
turkey vegetable	9⅜ oz	40	6	150
vegetable	10¾ oz	60	4	140
	9½ oz	40	4	130
vegetable, Mediterranean	9½ oz	60	5	160

CONDENSED SOUPS, AS PACKAGED

	Portion	Calcium (mg)	Total Fat (g)	Total Calor
asparagus, cream of	4 oz	20	4	90
bean w/bacon	4 oz	60	5	150
beef broth (bouillon)	4 oz	<20	0	16
beef noodle	4 oz	<20	3	70
black bean	4 oz	20	2	110
celery, cream of	4 oz	20	7	100
cheddar cheese	4 oz	80	8	130
chicken, cream of	4 oz	20	7	110
chicken & dumplings	4 oz	<20	3	80
chicken broth	4 oz	<20	2	35
chicken gumbo	4 oz	20	2	60
chicken noodle	4 oz	<20	2	70
chicken vegetable	4 oz	<20	3	70
chicken w/rice	4 oz	<20	2	60
chili beef	4 oz	20	5	130
clam chowder (Manhattan style)	4 oz	20	2	70
clam chowder (New England style)	4 oz	20	3	80
prepared w/whole milk	4 oz	150	7	150
French onion	4 oz	20	2	60
green pea	4 oz	<20	3	160
minestrone	4 oz	20	2	80
mushroom, cream of	4 oz	20	7	100
mushroom, Golden	4 oz	<20	3	80
nacho cheese	4 oz	100	8	100
noodles & ground beef	4 oz	<20	4	90
onion, cream of	4 oz	20	5	100
prepared w/whole milk	4 oz	80	7	140

	Portion	Calcium (mg)	Total Fat (g)	Total Calor
oyster stew	4 oz	<20	5	80
prepared w/whole milk	4 oz	100	9	150
pepper pot	4 oz	<20	4	90
potato, cream of	4 oz	<20	3	70
prepared w/whole milk	4 oz	20	4	110
Scotch broth	4 oz	<20	3	80
shrimp, cream of	4 oz	<20	6	90
prepared w/whole milk	4 oz	150	10	160
Spanish-style vegetable (gazpacho)	4 oz	20	0	45
split pea w/ham & bacon	4 oz	<20	4	160
tomato	4 oz	<20	2	90
prepared w/whole milk	4 oz	100	6	160
tomato bisque	4 oz	20	3	120
tomato rice, Old Fashioned	4 oz	<20	2	110
turkey noodle	4 oz	<20	3	70
turkey vegetable	4 oz	<20	3	70
vegetable	4 oz	<20	2	90
vegetable, Old Fashioned	4 oz	<20	2	60
vegetable, vegetarian	4 oz	<20	2	90
vegetable beef	4 oz	<20	2	70
won ton	4 oz	<20	1	40

CREAMY NATURAL SOUPS, CONDENSED

	Portion	Calcium (mg)	Total Fat (g)	Total Calor
asparagus, prepared w/whole milk	4 oz	100	9	170
potato, prepared w/whole milk	4 oz	100	11	190

DRY SOUP MIXES, AS PACKAGED

	Portion	Calcium (mg)	Total Fat (g)	Total Calor
cheddar cheese	1 oz	200	10	160
chicken noodle	1 oz	<20	2	100
chicken rice	1 oz	<20	2	90
noodle	1 oz	<20	2	110
onion	½ oz	20	0	50
onion mushroom	½ oz	<20	0	50

HOME COOKIN' SOUPS, READY-TO-SERVE

	Portion	Calcium (mg)	Total Fat (g)	Total Calor
chicken w/noodles	10¾ oz	40	4	140
country vegetable	10¾ oz	60	2	120
lentil	10¾ oz	40	1	170
minestrone	10¾ oz	60	3	140
split pea w/ham	10¾ oz	40	4	210
vegetable beef	10¾ oz	40	3	150

LOW-SODIUM SOUPS, READY-TO-SERVE

	Portion	Calcium (mg)	Total Fat (g)	Total Calor
beef & mushroom, chunky	10¾ oz	40	7	210
chicken broth	10½ oz	<20	2	40
chicken vegetable, chunky	10¾ oz	40	11	240
chicken w/noodles	10¾ oz	20	5	160
French onion	10½ oz	20	4	80

	Portion	Calcium (mg)	Total Fat (g)	Total Calor
mushroom, cream of	10½ oz	60	14	200
split pea	10¾ oz	40	5	240
tomato w/tomato pieces	10½ oz	40	5	180
vegetable beef, chunky	10¾ oz	40	5	170

SEMICONDENSED SOUPS, AS PREPARED

bean w/ham, Old Fashioned	11 oz	80	7	220
chicken & noodles, Golden	11 oz	20	4	120
clam chowder (New England)	11 oz	60	4	130
prepared w/whole milk	11 oz	150	7	190
mushroom, savory cream of	11 oz	20	13	180
Tomato Royale	11 oz	20	3	180
vegetable, Old World	11 oz	60	4	130
vegetable beef & bacon, Burly	11 oz	60	5	160

College Inn
beef broth	1 c	<20	0	18
chicken broth	1 c	<20	3	35

Health Valley
bean, regular or no salt	4 oz	52	3	115
beef broth, regular or no salt	4 oz	3	0	10
chicken broth, regular or no salt	4 oz	4	2	30
clam chowder, regular or no salt	4 oz	40	3	80
green split pea				
regular	4 oz	9	0	70
no salt	4 oz	9	1	80
lentil, regular or no salt	4 oz	7	4	80
minestrone, regular or no salt	4 oz	7	4	90
minestrone, chunky				
regular	4 oz	33	1	70
no salt	4 oz	20	1	70
mushroom, regular or no salt	4 oz	53	3	70
potato, regular or no salt	4 oz	112	2	70
tomato, regular or no salt	4 oz	4	2	60
vegetable, regular or no salt	4 oz	6	4	80
vegetable, chunky				
regular	4 oz	33	2	70
no salt	4 oz	20	2	70
vegetable chicken, chunky				
regular	4 oz	31	7	120
no salt	4 oz	19	7	120

Nissin
CUP O'NOODLES
beef	1 pkg = 1 c	20	14	290
chicken	1 pkg = 1 c	20	16	300
shrimp	1 pkg = 1 c	20	14	300

	Portion	Calcium (mg)	Total Fat (g)	Total Calor
HEARTY CUP O'NOODLES				
cream of chicken	1 pkg = 1 c	40	17	330
OODLES OF NOODLES				
beef	1 pkg = 1 c	20	18	390
chicken	1 pkg = 1 c	20	18	400
QUICK 'N TENDER				
chicken	1 pkg = 1 c	100	28	600
STIR 'N READY				
chicken	1 pkg = 1 c	20	10	190
TWIN CUP O'NOODLES				
chicken	1 pkg = 1 c	<20	7	150
Rokeach *CONDENSED SOUPS*				
celery, cream of	5 oz	6	4	90
mushroom, cream of	5 oz	6	10	150
tomato	5 oz	2	1	90
tomato w/rice	5 oz	4	5	160
vegetarian vegetable	5 oz	2	3	90
READY-TO-SERVE SOUPS				
borscht	8 fl oz	11	tr	96
Stouffer's Frozen Soups				
clam chowder (New England)	8 oz	80	11	200
spinach, cream of	8 oz	200	14	220
split pea w/ham	8¼ oz	20	3	200
Swanson				
beef broth	7¼ oz	<20	1	20
chicken broth	7¼ oz	<20	2	30

❏ **SOUR CREAM** *See* MILK, MILK SUBSTITUTES, & MILK PRODUCTS

❏ **SOYBEANS & SOYBEAN PRODUCTS**

Soybeans

boiled	½ c	88	8	149
dry roasted	½ c	232	19	387
mature seeds, sprouted				
raw	½ c	24	2	45

	Portion	Calcium (mg)	Total Fat (g)	Total Calor
mature seeds, sprouted *(cont.)*				
steamed	½ c	28	2	38
stir-fried	3½ oz	82	7	125
roasted	½ c	119	22	405

Soybean Products

	Portion	Calcium (mg)	Total Fat (g)	Total Calor
fermented products				
miso	½ c	92	8	284
natto	½ c	191	10	187
tempeh	½ c	77	6	165
soy flour				
full-fat				
raw	½ c stirred	87	9	182
roasted	½ c stirred	79	9	184
low-fat	½ c stirred	83	3	163
defatted	½ c stirred	120	1	164
soy meal, defatted, raw	½ c	149	1	206
soy milk, fluid	1 c	10	5	79
soy protein				
concentrate	1 oz	102	tr	92
isolate	1 oz	50	1	94
soy sauce				
made from hydrolyzed vege-	1 T	1	tr	7
table protein	¼ c	3	tr	24
made from soy (tamari)	1 T	4	tr	11
	¼ c	12	tr	35
made from soy & wheat	1 T	3	tr	9
(shoyu)	¼ c	10	tr	30
teriyaki sauce				
dehydrated	1 pkt = 1.6 oz	112	1	130
prepared w/water	1 c	112	1	131
ready-to-serve	1 T	4	0	15
	1 fl oz	9	0	30
tofu				
raw				
regular, made w/nigari	4.1 oz	122	6	88
	½ c	130	6	94
regular, made w/calcium	4.1 oz	406	6	88
sulfate	½ c	434	6	94
firm, made w/nigari	2.9 oz	166	7	118
	½ c	258	11	183
firm, made w/calcium sul-	2.9 oz	553	7	118
fate	½ c	860	11	183
dried-frozen (koyadofu)				
prepared w/nigari	0.6 oz	62	5	82
prepared w/calcium sulfate	0.6 oz	363	5	82
fried				
prepared w/nigari	½ oz	48	3	35
prepared w/calcium sulfate	½ oz	125	3	35

	Portion	Calcium (mg)	Total Fat (g)	Total Calor
okara	½ c	49	1	47
salted & fermented (fuyu)				
prepared w/nigari	0.4 oz	5	1	13
prepared w/calcium sulfate	0.4 oz	135	1	13

▪ BRAND NAME

Arrowhead Mills				
soybean flakes	2 oz	100	11	250
soybeans	2 oz	150	10	230
soy flour	2 oz	100	11	250
Chun King				
soy sauce	1 t	<20	0	6
Fearn				
lecithin granules	2 level T	<20	12	100
liquid lecithin				
regular	1 T	<20	16	130
mint-flavored	1 T	<20	16	113
natural soya powder	¼ c	40	5	100
soya granules	¼ c	100	tr	140
soya protein isolate	¼ c	<20	tr	60
Health Valley				
Soy Moo soybean milk	8 fl oz	40	6	140
Kikkoman				
soy sauce, regular or lite	1 T	about 3	tr	10
stir-fry sauce	1 t	tr	tr	6
sweet & sour sauce	1 T	tr	tr	18
teriyaki sauce	1 T	about 5	tr	15

❏ SPICES *See* SEASONINGS

❏ STUFFINGS *See* BREADCRUMBS, CROUTONS, STUFFINGS, & SEASONED COATINGS

❏ SUGARS & SWEETENERS: HONEY, MOLASSES, SUGAR, SUGAR SUBSTITUTES, SYRUP, & TREACLE

HONEY

honey	1 T	1	0	61
	5 T	20	0	306

	Portion	Calcium (mg)	Total Fat (g)	Total Calor
MOLASSES				
first extraction, light	1 T	33	0	50
	5 T	165	0	252
second extraction, medium	1 T	58	0	46
	5 T	290	0	232
third extraction, blackstrap	1 T	116	0	43
	5 T	579	0	213
SUGAR				
brown	1 T	11	0	52
	5 T	53	0	364
maple	1 T	27	0	52
sugarcane juice	1 T	3	tr	16
white				
granulated	1 cube	tr	0	24
	1 t	tr	0	16
	1 T	tr	0	46
	½ c	5	0	385
powdered	1 T	?	0	42
	9 T	?	0	385
SYRUP				
cane	1 T	12	0	53
	5 T	60	0	263
corn	1 T	9	0	57
	5 T	46	0	287
dark corn	1 T	?	0	60
maple	1 T	33	0	50
	5 T	104	0	252
maple, imitation	1 T	2	0	55
	5 T	10	0	275
sorghum, pancake	1 T	30	0	52
table blend, pancake				
cane & maple	1 T	3	0	50
mainly corn	1 T	9	0	57
	5 T	46	0	286
TREACLE				
black	1 T	99	0	53
	5 T	495	0	265

▪ BRAND NAME

Aunt Jemima
| syrup | 1 fl oz | 0 | 0 | 103 |

	Portion	Calcium (mg)	Total Fat (g)	Total Calor
Butter Lite syrup	1 fl oz	0	0	52
Lite syrup	1 fl oz	0	0	60
Brer Rabbit				
molasses, light or dark	1 T	40	0	60
Diamond Crystal				
sugar substitute	1 pkg	2	0	1
Equal				
sugar substitute	1 pkg	0	0	4
Golden Griddle				
syrup	1 T	<20	0	50
Grandma's Molasses				
gold label	1 T	22	0	70
green label	1 T	41	0	70
Karo				
corn syrup, dark or light	1 T	<20	0	60
pancake syrup	1 T	<20	0	60
Log Cabin				
syrup	1 fl oz	6	0	104
buttered syrup	1 fl oz	5	1	105
Country Kitchen syrup	1 fl oz	11	0	101
maple honey syrup	1 fl oz	7	0	106
NutraSweet				
sugar substitute	1 pkg	0	0	4
Sprinkle Sweet				
sugar substitute	⅛ t	?	0	2
Sugartwin				
sugar substitute				
white	1 pkg	8	0	3
white/brown	1 t	4	0	1
Sweet & Low				
sugar substitute	1 pkg	?	0	4
Sweet 10				
sugar substitute	⅛ t	?	0	0
Vermont Maid				
syrup	1 T	<20	0	50

❑ **SYRUP** *See* SUGARS & SWEETENERS

❑ **SYRUP, DESSERT** *See* DESSERT SAUCES, SYRUPS, & TOPPINGS

❑ **TOFU, FROZEN** *See* DESSERTS, FROZEN

	Portion	Calcium (mg)	Total Fat (g)	Total Calor

❑ **TREACLE** *See* SUGARS & SWEETENERS

❑ **TURKEY** *See* POULTRY, FRESH
& PROCESSED; PROCESSED MEAT
& POULTRY PRODUCTS

❑ **VEAL** *See* LAMB, VEAL,
& MISCELLANEOUS MEATS

❑ **VEGETABLES, PLAIN & PREPARED**
See also LEGUMES & LEGUME PRODUCTS; PICKLES,
OLIVES, RELISHES, & CHUTNEYS; RICE & GRAINS, PLAIN
& PREPARED

Vegetables, Plain

	Portion	Calcium (mg)	Total Fat (g)	Total Calor
alfalfa seeds *See* SEEDS & SEED-BASED BUTTERS, FLOURS, & MEALS				
amaranth				
raw	1 c	60	tr	7
boiled, drained	½ c	138	tr	14
arrowhead				
raw	1 medium corm = 0.4 oz	1	tr	12
boiled, drained	1 medium corm = 1.4 oz	1	tr	9
artichokes, globe & French varieties				
boiled	1 medium = 4.2 oz	47	tr	53
	½ c hearts	33	tr	37
frozen, boiled, drained	9 oz pkg	50	1	108
artichokes, Jerusalem *See* Jerusalem artichokes, *below*				
asparagus, cuts & spears				
raw	4 spears = 2 oz	12	tr	13
boiled	4 spears = 2.1 oz	15	tr	15
canned				
drained solids	½ c	?	1	24
solids & liquids	½ c	17	tr	17
frozen, boiled, drained	10 oz pkg	68	1	82
	4 spears = 2.1 oz	14	tr	17

	Portion	Calcium (mg)	Total Fat (g)	Total Calor
asparagus beans *See* yardlong beans, *under* LEGUMES & LEGUME PRODUCTS				
balsam pear				
leafy tips				
raw	½ c	20	tr	7
boiled, drained	½ c	12	tr	10
pods				
raw	1 c	18	tr	16
boiled, drained	½ c	6	tr	12
bamboo shoots				
raw	½ c	10	tr	21
boiled, drained	1 c	14	tr	15
canned, drained solids	1 c	10	1	25
basella *See* vinespinach, *below*				
beans, shellie, canned, solids & liquids	½ c	36	tr	37
beans, snap				
raw	½ c	21	tr	17
boiled, drained	½ c	29	tr	22
canned				
drained solids	½ c	18	tr	13
solids & liquids	½ c	29	tr	18
solids & liquids, seasoned	½ c	25	tr	18
frozen, boiled, drained	½ c	31	tr	18
beet greens				
raw	½ c	23	tr	4
boiled, drained	½ c	82	tr	20
beets				
raw	½ c sliced	11	tr	30
boiled, drained	½ c sliced	9	tr	26
canned				
drained solids	½ c sliced	?	tr	27
solids & liquids	½ c sliced	17	tr	36
pickled, canned, solids & liquids	½ c	13	tr	75
beets, Harvard, canned, solids & liquids	½ c sliced	13	tr	89
bittergourd; bittermelon *See* balsam pear, *above*				
bok choy *See* cabbage, Chinese, *below*				
borage				
raw	½ c	41	tr	9
boiled, drained	3½ oz	102	1	25
broad beans *See* LEGUMES & LEGUME PRODUCTS				
broccoli				
raw	1 spear = 5.3 oz	73	1	42
boiled, drained	½ c	89	tr	23
	1 spear = 6.3 oz	205	1	53
frozen, boiled, drained	½ c chopped	47	tr	25
	½ c spears	127	tr	69
	10 oz pkg spears	47	tr	25

	Portion	Calcium (mg)	Total Fat (g)	Total Calor
brussels sprouts				
boiled, drained	1 sprout = 0.73 oz	7	tr	8
	½ c	28	tr	30
frozen, boiled, drained	½ c	19	tr	33
burdock root				
raw	1 c	48	tr	85
	5½ oz	64	tr	112
boiled, drained	1 c	62	tr	110
	5.8 oz	82	tr	146
butterbur				
raw	1 c	97	tr	13
boiled, drained	3½ oz	59	tr	8
cabbage				
raw	½ c shredded	16	tr	8
boiled, drained	½ c shredded	25	tr	16
cabbage, Chinese				
bok choy				
raw	½ c shredded	37	tr	5
boiled, drained	½ c shredded	79	tr	10
pe-tsai				
raw	½ c shredded	29	tr	6
boiled, drained	1 c shredded	38	tr	16
cabbage, red				
raw	½ c shredded	18	tr	10
boiled, drained	½ c shredded	28	tr	16
cabbage, savoy				
raw	½ c shredded	12	tr	10
boiled, drained	½ c shredded	22	tr	18
cardoon, raw	½ c shredded	62	tr	18
carrots				
raw	½ c shredded	15	tr	24
	2½ oz	19	tr	31
boiled, drained	½ c sliced	24	tr	35
	1.6 oz	14	tr	21
canned				
drained solids	½ c sliced	19	tr	17
solids & liquids	½ c sliced	31	tr	28
frozen, boiled, drained	½ c sliced	21	tr	26
cassava, raw	3½ oz	91	tr	120
cauliflower				
raw	½ c pieces	14	tr	12
	3 flowerets = 2 oz	16	tr	13
boiled, drained	½ c pieces	17	tr	15
frozen, boiled, drained	½ c pieces	15	tr	17
celeriac				
raw	½ c	34	tr	31
boiled, drained	3½ oz	26	tr	25

	Portion	Calcium (mg)	Total Fat (g)	Total Calor
celery				
raw	1 stalk = 1.4 oz	14	tr	6
	½ c diced	22	tr	9
boiled, drained	½ c diced	27	tr	11
celtuce, raw	1 leaf = 0.3 oz	3	tr	2
chard, Swiss				
raw	½ c chopped	9	tr	3
boiled, drained	½ c chopped	51	tr	18
chayote, fruit				
raw	1 c pieces	25	tr	32
	7.1 oz	39	1	49
boiled, drained	1 c pieces	21	1	38
chicory, raw				
greens	½ c chopped	90	tr	21
roots	½ c pieces	18	tr	33
witloof	½ c	?	tr	7
Chinese parsley See coriander, below				
Chinese preserving melon See wax gourd, below				
chives				
raw	1 t	1	tr	0
raw	1 T	2	tr	1
freeze-dried	1 T	2	tr	1
chrysanthemum, garland				
raw	1 c pieces	14	tr	4
boiled, drained	½ c pieces	34	tr	10
collards				
raw	½ c chopped	109	tr	18
boiled, drained	½ c chopped	74	tr	13
frozen, boiled, drained	½ c chopped	179	tr	31
coriander (cilantro), raw	¼ c	4	tr	1
corn, sweet				
raw	½ c kernels	2	1	66
	kernels from 1 ear	2	1	77
boiled, drained	½ c kernels	2	1	89
	kernels from 1 ear	2	1	83
canned				
cream style	½ c	4	1	93
in brine, drained solids	½ c	?	1	66
in brine, solids & liquids	½ c	5	1	79
vacuum pack	½ c	5	1	83
w/red & green peppers, solids & liquids	½ c	5	1	86
frozen, boiled, drained	½ c kernels	2	tr	67
	kernels from 1 ear	2	tr	59

cowpeas See LEGUMES & LEGUME PRODUCTS

	Portion	Calcium (mg)	Total Fat (g)	Total Calor
cress, garden				
raw	1 sprig	1	tr	0
	½ c	20	tr	8
boiled, drained	½ c	41	tr	16
cucumber, raw	½ c sliced	7	tr	7
	10½ oz	42	tr	39
daikon *See* radishes: Oriental, *below*				
dandelion greens				
raw	½ c chopped	52	tr	13
boiled, drained	½ c chopped	73	tr	17
dasheen *See* taro, *below*				
dock				
raw	½ c chopped	29	tr	15
boiled, drained	3½ oz	38	1	20
eggplant, boiled, drained	1 c cubed	5	tr	27
endive, raw	½ c chopped	13	tr	4
endive, Belgian *See* chicory: witloof, *above*				
eppaw, raw	½ c	55	1	75
escarole *See* endive, *above*				
garlic, raw	1 clove = 0.1 oz	5	tr	4
ginger root, raw	0.4 oz	2	tr	8
	¼ c sliced	4	tr	17
gourd				
dishcloth, boiled, drained	½ c	8	tr	50
white-flowered (calabash), boiled, drained	½ c cubed	18	tr	11
horseradish-tree				
leafy tips				
raw	½ c chopped	?	tr	6
boiled, drained	½ c chopped	?	tr	13
pods				
raw	1 pod = 0.4 oz	3	tr	4
boiled, drained	½ c sliced	12	tr	21
hyacinth beans *See* LEGUMES & LEGUME PRODUCTS				
Jerusalem artichokes, raw	½ c sliced	16	tr	57
jicama *See* yam bean, *below*				
jute (pot herb), boiled, drained	½ c	91	tr	16
kale				
raw	½ c chopped	46	tr	17
boiled, drained	½ c chopped	47	tr	21
frozen, boiled, drained	½ c chopped	90	tr	20
kale, Scotch				
raw	½ c chopped	70	tr	14
boiled, drained	½ c chopped	86	tr	18
kanpyo (dried gourd strips)	0.7 oz	53	tr	49
kohlrabi				
raw	½ c sliced	17	tr	19
boiled, drained	½ c sliced	20	tr	24

	Portion	Calcium (mg)	Total Fat (g)	Total Calor
lamb's-quarters, boiled, drained	½ c chopped	232	1	29
leeks				
raw	¼ c chopped	15	tr	16
boiled, drained	¼ c chopped	8	tr	8
freeze-dried	1 T	1	0	1
lentils *See* LEGUMES & LEGUME PRODUCTS				
lettuce, raw				
butterhead (includes Boston & Bibb types)	2 leaves = ½ oz	?	tr	2
	1 head = 5.7 oz	?	tr	21
cos or romaine	1 inner leaf = 0.35 oz	4	tr	2
	½ c shredded	10	tr	4
iceberg	1 leaf = 0.7 oz	4	tr	3
	1 head = 1 lb 3 oz	102	1	70
looseleaf	1 leaf = 0.35 oz	7	tr	2
	½ c shredded	19	tr	5
lima beans *See* LEGUMES & LEGUME PRODUCTS				
lotus root, boiled, drained	3.1 oz	23	tr	59
manioc *See* cassava, *above*				
mountain yam, Hawaii, steamed	½ c	5	tr	59
mung beans *See* LEGUMES & LEGUME PRODUCTS				
mushrooms				
raw	½ c pieces	2	tr	9
boiled, drained	½ c pieces	4	tr	21
canned, drained solids	½ c pieces	?	tr	19
mushrooms, shitake				
dried	0.1 oz	0	tr	11
cooked	½ oz	2	tr	40
mustard greens				
raw	½ c chopped	29	tr	7
boiled, drained	½ c chopped	52	tr	11
frozen, boiled, drained	½ c chopped	75	tr	14
mustard spinach				
raw	½ c chopped	158	tr	17
boiled, drained	½ c chopped	142	tr	14
New Zealand spinach				
raw	½ c chopped	16	tr	4
boiled, drained	½ c chopped	43	tr	11
okra				
boiled, drained	½ c sliced	50	tr	25
frozen, boiled, drained	½ c sliced	88	tr	34
onions				
raw	1 T chopped	2	tr	3
	½ c chopped	20	tr	27

	Portion	Calcium (mg)	Total Fat (g)	Total Calor
onions *(cont.)*				
boiled, drained	1 T chopped	4	tr	4
	½ c chopped	29	tr	29
canned, solids & liquids	2.2 oz	29	tr	12
dehydrated flakes	1 T	13	tr	16
frozen, boiled, drained	1 T chopped	2	tr	4
	½ c chopped	17	tr	30
onions, spring, raw	1 T chopped	4	tr	2
	½ c chopped	30	tr	13
onions, Welsh, raw	3½ oz	18	tr	34
oysterplant *See* salsify, *below*				
parsley				
raw	10 sprigs = 0.35 oz	13	tr	3
	½ c chopped	39	tr	10
freeze-dried	1 T	1	tr	1
parsnips				
raw	½ c sliced	24	tr	50
boiled, drained	½ c sliced	29	tr	63
peas, edible pods				
raw	½ c	31	tr	30
boiled, drained	½ c	33	tr	34
frozen, boiled, drained	½ c	48	tr	42
	10 oz pkg	150	1	132
peas, green				
raw	½ c	19	tr	63
boiled, drained	½ c	22	tr	67
canned				
drained solids	½ c	17	tr	59
solids & liquids	½ c	22	tr	61
solids & liquids, seasoned	½ c	18	tr	57
frozen, boiled, drained	½ c	19	tr	63
peas, mature seeds, sprouted				
raw	½ c	21	tr	77
boiled, drained	3½ oz	26	1	118
peas, split *See* split peas, *under* LEGUMES & LEGUME PRODUCTS				
peas & carrots				
canned, solids & liquids	½ c	29	tr	48
frozen, boiled, drained	½ c	18	tr	38
	10 oz pkg	64	1	133
peas & onions				
canned, solids & liquids	½ c	10	tr	30
frozen, boiled, drained	½ c	13	tr	40
pepeao				
raw	0.2 oz	1	0	2
dried	½ c	14	tr	36
peppers				
hot chili				
raw	1 pepper = 1.6 oz	8	tr	18
	½ c chopped	13	tr	30

	Portion	Calcium (mg)	Total Fat (g)	Total Calor
canned, solids & liquids	1 pepper = 2.6 oz	5	tr	18
	½ c chopped	5	tr	17
jalapeño, canned, solids & liquids	½ c chopped	18	tr	17
sweet				
raw	1 pepper = 2.6 oz	4	tr	18
	½ c chopped	3	tr	12
boiled, drained	1 pepper = 2.6 oz	3	tr	13
	½ c chopped	3	tr	12
canned, solids & liquids	½ c halves	28	tr	13
freeze-dried	1 T	1	tr	1
	¼ c	2	tr	5
frozen, unprepared, chopped	10 oz pkg	26	1	58
frozen, boiled, drained	3½ oz chopped	8	tr	18
pigeon peas *See* LEGUMES & LEGUME PRODUCTS				
pimientos *See* PICKLES, OLIVES, RELISHES, & CHUTNEYS				
pinto beans *See* LEGUMES & LEGUME PRODUCTS				
poi	½ c	19	tr	134
pokeberry shoots				
raw	½ c	42	tr	18
boiled, drained	½ c	43	tr	16
potatoes				
raw				
flesh	3.9 oz	8	tr	88
skin	1.3 oz	11	tr	22
baked				
flesh & skin	7.1 oz	20	tr	220
flesh	5½ oz	8	tr	145
skin	2 oz	20	tr	115
boiled in skin				
flesh	4.8 oz	7	tr	119
skin	1.2 oz	15	tr	27
boiled w/out skin, flesh	4.8 oz	10	tr	116
canned				
drained solids	1.2 oz	2	tr	21
solids & liquids	1 c	89	tr	120
frozen, whole, unprepared	½ c	7	tr	71
microwaved in skin				
flesh & skin	7.1 oz	22	tr	212
flesh	5½ oz	8	tr	156
skin	2 oz	27	tr	77
pumpkin				
boiled, drained	½ c mashed	18	tr	24
canned	½ c	32	tr	41
pumpkin flowers				
raw	1 c	13	tr	5
boiled, drained	½ c	25	tr	10

	Portion	Calcium (mg)	Total Fat (g)	Total Calor
pumpkin leaves, boiled, drained	½ c	15	tr	7
purslane				
raw	1 c	28	tr	7
boiled, drained	1 c	90	tr	21
radishes, raw	10 radishes = 1.6 oz	9	tr	7
Oriental				
raw	½ c	12	tr	8
boiled, drained	½ c sliced	12	tr	13
dried	½ c	365	tr	157
white icicle, raw	½ c sliced	14	tr	7
radish seeds, sprouted, raw	½ c	10	tr	8
rutabagas				
raw	½ c cubed	33	tr	25
boiled, drained	½ c cubed	36	tr	29
	½ c mashed	50	tr	41
salsify				
raw	½ c sliced	40	tr	55
boiled, drained	½ c sliced	32	tr	46
seaweed				
agar, raw	3½ oz	54	tr	26
kelp, raw	3½ oz	168	1	43
laver, raw	3½ oz	70	tr	35
spirulina				
raw	3½ oz	?	tr	26
dried	3½ oz	?	8	290
wakame, raw	3½ oz	150	1	45
sesbania flower				
raw	1 c	4	tr	5
steamed	1 c	23	tr	23
shallots				
raw	1 T chopped	4	tr	7
freeze-dried	1 T	2	tr	3
snow peas *See* peas, edible pods, *above*				
soybeans *See* SOYBEANS & SOYBEAN PRODUCTS				
spinach				
raw	½ c chopped	28	tr	6
boiled, drained	½ c	122	tr	21
canned				
drained solids	½ c	135	1	25
solids & liquids	½ c	97	tr	22
frozen, boiled, drained	½ c	139	tr	27
	10 oz pkg	321	tr	63
spinach, mustard *See* mustard spinach, *above*				
spinach, New Zealand *See* New Zealand spinach, *above*				
split peas *See* LEGUMES & LEGUME PRODUCTS				
sprouts *See* plant name (alfalfa, mung bean, etc.)				
squash, summer				
all varieties				
raw	½ c sliced	13	tr	13

	Portion	Calcium (mg)	Total Fat (g)	Total Calor
boiled, drained	½ c sliced	24	tr	18
crookneck				
raw	½ c sliced	14	tr	12
boiled, drained	½ c sliced	24	tr	18
canned, drained solids	½ c sliced	13	tr	14
frozen, boiled, drained	½ c sliced	19	tr	24
scallop				
raw	½ c sliced	12	tr	12
boiled, drained	½ c sliced	14	tr	14
zucchini				
raw	½ c sliced	10	tr	9
boiled, drained	½ c sliced	12	tr	14
canned, Italian style, in tomato sauce	½ c	19	tr	33
frozen, boiled, drained	½ c	19	tr	19
squash, winter				
all varieties				
raw	½ c cubed	18	tr	21
baked	½ c cubed	14	1	39
acorn				
baked	½ c cubed	45	tr	57
boiled	½ c mashed	32	tr	41
butternut				
baked	½ c cubed	42	tr	41
frozen, boiled	½ c mashed	23	tr	47
hubbard				
baked	½ c cubed	17	1	51
boiled	½ c mashed	12	tr	35
spaghetti, boiled, drained, baked	½ c	17	tr	23
string beans *See* beans, snap, *above*				
succotash				
boiled, drained	½ c	16	1	111
canned				
w/cream-style corn	½ c	15	1	102
w/whole kernel corn, solids & liquids	½ c	14	1	81
frozen, boiled, drained	½ c	13	1	79
swamp cabbage				
raw	1 c chopped	43	tr	11
boiled, drained	1 c chopped	53	tr	20
sweet potatoes				
baked in skin	½ c mashed	28	tr	103
	1 potato = 4 oz	32	tr	118
boiled w/out skin	½ c mashed	35	tr	172
candied	3.7 oz	27	3	144
canned				
in syrup, drained solids	1 c	32	1	213
in syrup, solids & liquids	1 c	35	tr	202

	Portion	Calcium (mg)	Total Fat (g)	Total Calor
sweet potatoes: canned *(cont.)*				
mashed	1 c	76	1	258
vacuum packed	1 c pieces	44	tr	183
	1 c mashed	56	1	233
frozen, baked	½ c cubed	31	tr	88
sweet potato leaves				
raw	1 c chopped	13	tr	12
steamed	1 c	15	tr	22
Swiss chard *See* chard, Swiss, *above*				
taro				
raw	½ c sliced	22	tr	56
cooked	½ c sliced	12	tr	94
taro chips	10 chips = 0.8 oz	10	6	110
taro leaves				
raw	1 c	30	tr	12
steamed	1 c	124	1	35
taro shoots				
raw	1 shoot = 2.9 oz	10	tr	9
cooked	½ c sliced	9	tr	10
taro, Tahitian				
raw	½ c sliced	80	1	25
cooked	½ c sliced	101	tr	30
tomatoes, green, raw	1 tomato = 4.3 oz	16	tr	30
tomatoes, red, ripe				
raw	1 tomato = 4.3 oz	8	tr	24
boiled	½ c	10	tr	30
canned				
stewed	½ c	42	tr	34
wedges in juice	½ c	34	tr	34
w/green chilies	½ c	24	tr	18
whole	½ c	32	tr	24
stewed	1 c	19	2	59
tomato paste, canned	½ c	46	1	110
tomato puree, canned	1 c	37	tr	102
tomato sauce *See* SAUCES, GRAVIES, & CONDIMENTS				
towel gourd *See* gourd: dishcloth, *above*				
tree fern, cooked	½ c chopped	6	tr	28
turnip greens				
raw	½ c chopped	53	tr	7
boiled, drained	½ c chopped	99	tr	15
canned, solids & liquids	½ c	138	tr	17
frozen, boiled, drained	½ c	125	tr	24
turnip greens & turnips, frozen, boiled, drained	3½ oz	91	tr	17
turnips				
raw	½ c cubed	20	tr	18
boiled, drained	½ c cubed	18	tr	14
frozen, boiled, drained	3½ oz	32	tr	23

	Portion	Calcium (mg)	Total Fat (g)	Total Calor
vegetables, mixed				
canned				
drained solids	½ c	22	tr	39
solids & liquids	½ c	26	tr	44
frozen, boiled, drained	½ c	22	tr	54
	10 oz pkg	67	tr	163
vinespinach, raw	3½ oz	109	tr	19
water chestnuts, Chinese				
raw	1¼ oz	4	tr	38
canned, solids & liquids	1 oz	1	tr	14
watercress, raw	½ c chopped	20	tr	2
wax beans See beans, snap, *above*				
wax gourd (Chinese preserving melon), boiled, drained	½ c cubed	16	tr	11
winged beans See LEGUMES & LEGUME PRODUCTS				
yam, baked or boiled	½ c cubed	9	tr	79
yam bean (tuber only)				
raw	1 c sliced	18	tr	49
boiled, drained	3½ oz	16	tr	46
yardlong beans See LEGUMES & LEGUME PRODUCTS				

Vegetables, Prepared

	Portion	Calcium (mg)	Total Fat (g)	Total Calor
coleslaw	½ c	27	2	42
corn pudding	1 c	100	13	271
onion rings, breaded, frozen, heated in oven	0.7 oz	6	5	81
potato chips & sticks See SNACKS				
potatoes, au gratin				
dry mix, prepared	5½ oz pkg	682	34	764
homemade	½ c	146	9	160
potatoes, french fried, frozen				
fried in animal fat & vegetable oil	1.8 oz	10	8	158
fried in vegetable oil	1.8 oz	10	8	158
heated in oven	1.8 oz	4	4	111
cottage-cut, heated in oven	1.8 oz	5	4	109
extruded, heated in oven	1.8 oz	6	9	163
potatoes, hashed brown				
frozen, plain, prepared	½ c	12	9	170
frozen, w/butter sauce, unprepared	6 oz pkg	43	11	229
homemade, prepared in vegetable oil	½ c	6	11	163
potatoes, mashed				
dehydrated flakes, prepared, whole milk & butter added	½ c	52	6	118
granules w/milk, prepared	½ c	33	2	83

	Portion	Calcium (mg)	Total Fat (g)	Total Calor
potatoes, mashed *(cont.)*				
granules w/out milk, prepared, whole milk & butter added	½ c	57	7	137
homemade w/whole milk & margarine	½ c	27	4	111
homemade w/whole milk	½ c	28	1	81
potatoes, O'Brien				
frozen, prepared	3½ oz	20	13	204
homemade	1 c	70	2	157
potatoes, scalloped				
dry mix, prepared w/whole milk & butter	5½ oz pkg	296	35	764
homemade	½ c	70	4	105
potato flour *See* FLOURS & CORNMEALS				
potato pancakes, homemade	2.7 oz	21	13	495
potato puffs, frozen, fried in vegetable oil	¼ oz	2	1	16
potato salad	½ c	24	10	179
sauerkraut, canned, solids & liquids	½ c	36	tr	22
spinach soufflé	1 c	230	18	218

• BRAND NAME

Arrowhead Mills				
potato flakes	2 oz	40	0	140
B&B				
mushrooms, canned	2 oz	0	<1	25
Birds Eye Frozen Vegetables *REGULAR*				
asparagus cuts	3.3 oz	20	0	25
beans				
baby lima	3.3 oz	40	0	130
cut or French cut green	3 oz	40	0	25
Italian green	3 oz	40	0	30
broccoli				
chopped	3.3 oz	40	0	25
cuts	3.3 oz	60	0	25
brussels sprouts	3.3 oz	20	0	35
cauliflower	3.3 oz	20	0	25
corn, sweet	3.3 oz	<20	1	80
corn on the cob	1 ear	<20	1	120
mixed vegetables	3.3 oz	20	0	60
onions, small whole	4 oz	40	0	40
peas, green	3.3 oz	20	0	80
spinach				
chopped	3.3 oz	100	0	20
whole leaf	3.3 oz	100	0	20

	Portion	Calcium (mg)	Total Fat (g)	Total Calor
squash, cooked, winter	4 oz	20	0	45
CHEESE SAUCE COMBINATIONS				
baby brussels sprouts w/ cheese sauce	4½ oz	80	6	110
broccoli w/cheese sauce	5 oz	100	6	120
broccoli w/creamy Italian cheese sauce	4½ oz	100	6	90
cauliflower w/cheese sauce	5 oz	80	6	110
peas & pearl onions w/ cheese sauce	5 oz	80	5	140
COMBINATION				
broccoli, carrots, pasta twists	3.3 oz	40	4	90
corn, green beans, pasta curls	3.3 oz	60	5	110
creamed spinach	3 oz	80	4	60
fresh green beans w/toasted almonds	3 oz	40	2	50
green peas & pearl onions	3.3 oz	<20	0	70
green peas & potatoes w/ cream sauce	2.6 oz	40	6	130
mixed vegetables w/onion sauce	2.6 oz	40	5	100
rice & green peas w/mush- rooms	2.3 oz	<20	0	110
small onions w/cream sauce	3 oz	60	6	110
DELUXE				
artichoke hearts	3 oz	<20	0	30
beans, whole green	3 oz	40	0	25
broccoli florets	3.3 oz	40	0	25
carrots, baby peas, & pearl onions	3.3 oz	20	0	50
carrots, whole baby	3.3 oz	20	0	40
corn, tender sweet	3.3 oz	<20	1	80
peas, tender tiny	3.3 oz	<20	0	60
FARM FRESH MIXTURES				
broccoli, baby carrots, water chestnuts	3.2 oz	40	0	35
broccoli, cauliflower, carrots	3.2 oz	40	0	25
broccoli, corn, red peppers	3.2 oz	20	0	50
broccoli, green beans, pearl onions, red peppers	3.2 oz	40	0	25
broccoli, red peppers, bam- boo shoots, straw mush- rooms	3.2 oz	40	0	25
brussels sprouts, cauliflower, carrots	3.2 oz	20	0	30

	Portion	Calcium (mg)	Total Fat (g)	Total Calor
cauliflower, baby whole carrots, snow pea pods	3.2 oz	20	0	30

INTERNATIONAL RECIPES

	Portion	Calcium (mg)	Total Fat (g)	Total Calor
Bavarian style	3.3 oz	40	6	110
Chinese style	3.3 oz	20	5	80
chow mein style	3.3 oz	20	4	90
Italian style	3.3 oz	40	7	110
Japanese style	3.3 oz	20	6	100
Mandarin style	3.3 oz	40	4	90
New England style	3.3 oz	20	7	130
pasta primavera style	3.3 oz	100	5	120
San Francisco style	3.3 oz	20	5	100

STIR-FRY

	Portion	Calcium (mg)	Total Fat (g)	Total Calor
Chinese style	3.3 oz	40	0	35
Japanese style	3.3 oz	20	0	30
Chun King				
bamboo shoots	2 oz	<20	0	16
bean sprouts	4 oz	20	0	40
chow mein vegetables	4 oz	20	0	35
water chestnuts, whole, sliced	2 oz	<20	0	45
Claussen				
sauerkraut	½ c	25	tr	17
Fresh Chef				
Holiday cole slaw	4 oz	20	15	200
Old Fashioned potato salad	4 oz	20	14	210
Joan of Arc				
garden salad	½ c	40	<1	80
potato salad				
German style	½ c	600	2	120
Home Style	½ c	0	9	160
pumpkin	½ c	60	2	50
sweet potatoes				
cut	½ c	0	<1	110
in orange pineapple sauce	½ c	20	<1	180
mashed	½ c	20	<1	130
whole, packed in heavy syrup	½ c	0	<1	150
wax beans, cut	½ c	100	<1	25
Le Sueur				
CANNED				
asparagus spears	½ c	0	0	30
whole kernel corn	½ c	0	0	80

	Portion	Calcium (mg)	Total Fat (g)	Total Calor
FROZEN, IN BUTTER SAUCE				
early peas	½ c	20	2	90
minipeas, pea pods, & water chestnuts	½ c	20	2	80
peas, onions, & carrots	½ c	0	3	80
Mexicorn				
Mexicorn w/peppers	½ c	0	0	80
Mrs. Paul's Prepared Vegetables				
candied yams	4 oz	20	1	200
corn fritters	2	20	12	250
eggplant parmigiana	5½ oz	100	17	270
fried eggplant sticks	3½ oz	20	12	240
onion rings, crispy	2½ oz	<20	10	180
zucchini sticks, light batter	3 oz	20	12	200
Ortega				
green chiles, whole, diced, strips, sliced	1 oz	<20	0	10
hot peppers, whole, diced	1 oz	<20	0	8
jalapeño peppers, whole, diced	1 oz	<20	0	10
tomatoes & jalapeños	1 oz	<20	0	8
Pepperidge Farm Vegetables in Pastry				
broccoli w/cheese	1	60	17	250
cauliflower & cheese sauce	1	60	13	210
Pillsbury				
BUTTER SAUCE VEGETABLES				
baby lima beans	½ c	20	2	110
broccoli cauliflower carrots	½ c	20	1	30
broccoli spears	½ c	20	2	45
brussels sprouts	½ c	20	1	60
cauliflower	½ c	20	1	30
cut green beans	½ c	20	1	35
cut leaf spinach	½ c	200	2	60
French-style green beans	½ c	20	1	40
mixed vegetables	½ c	20	2	80
Niblets corn	½ c	0	2	100
sweet peas	½ c	20	1	90
CANNED VEGETABLES				
asparagus cuts	½ c	0	0	20
cream-style corn	½ c	0	1	100
cut green beans	½ c	20	1	20
Golden Shoe Peg corn	½ c	0	1	90
mushrooms	2 oz	0	0	14
mushrooms in butter sauce	2 oz	0	<1	25
sweet peas	½ c	20	0	60
sweet peas & onions	½ c	20	<1	60
three bean salad	½ c	20	<1	80

	Portion	Calcium (mg)	Total Fat (g)	Total Calor
whole kernel corn, Vacuum Pak	½ c	0	0	90

CREAM & CHEESE SAUCE COMBINATION

	Portion	Calcium (mg)	Total Fat (g)	Total Calor
baby brussels sprouts in cheese-flavored sauce	½ c	60	2	80
broccoli cauliflower carrots in cheese-flavored sauce	½ c	60	2	70
broccoli in cheese-flavored sauce	½ c	60	2	70
broccoli in white cheddar cheese–flavored sauce	½ c	60	3	60
cauliflower in cheese-flavored sauce	½ c	60	2	60
cauliflower in white cheddar cheese–flavored sauce	½ c	60	3	70
creamed spinach	½ c	100	3	80
cream-style corn	½ c	0	1	120
peas in cream sauce	½ c	60	4	100

HARVEST FRESH

	Portion	Calcium (mg)	Total Fat (g)	Total Calor
broccoli spears	½ c	20	0	30
cut broccoli	½ c	20	0	25
cut green beans	½ c	20	0	20
early June peas	½ c	20	1	80
lima beans	½ c	20	1	70
mixed vegetables	½ c	20	0	45
Niblets corn	½ c	0	1	90
spinach	½ c	100	<1	40
sweet peas	½ c	20	0	60

HARVEST GET TOGETHERS

	Portion	Calcium (mg)	Total Fat (g)	Total Calor
Broccoli Cauliflower Medley	½ c	20	1	60
Broccoli Fanfare	½ c	20	1	70
Cauliflower Carrot Bonanza	½ c	0	3	60

POLYBAG VEGETABLES

	Portion	Calcium (mg)	Total Fat (g)	Total Calor
broccoli cuts	½ c	20	0	16
brussels sprouts	½ c	20	0	30
cauliflower cuts	½ c	0	0	12
green beans	½ c	20	0	20
lima beans	½ c	20	0	100
mixed vegetables	½ c	0	0	50
Niblets corn	½ c	0	1	80
Niblets corn on the cob	1 ear	0	1	150
sweet peas	½ c	0	0	60

	Portion	Calcium (mg)	Total Fat (g)	Total Calor
POTATO SIDE DISHES				
stuffed baked potato w/ cheese-flavored topping	1	40	6	200
stuffed baked potato w/sour cream & chives	1	40	10	230
VALLEY COMBINATION DUAL POUCH W/SAUCE				
American-style vegetables	½ c	0	2	90
Broccoli Cauliflower Medley	½ c	20	2	60
Broccoli Fanfare	½ c	20	2	80
Italian-style vegetables	½ c	40	2	50
Japanese-style vegetables	½ c	20	1	45
Le Sueur–style vegetables	½ c	20	2	90
Mexican-style vegetables	½ c	60	5	150
VALLEY COMBINATIONS, POLYBAG				
Broccoli Carrot Fanfare	½ c	20	0	20
Broccoli Cauliflower Supreme	½ c	20	0	18
Cauliflower Green Bean Festival	½ c	0	0	16
Corn Broccoli Bounty	½ c	0	1	45
Sweet Pea Cauliflower Medley	½ c	0	0	30
Stouffer				
broccoli in cheddar cheese sauce	4½ oz	150	10	150
corn soufflé	4 oz	40	7	150
creamed spinach	4½ oz	100	15	190
green bean mushroom casserole	4¾ oz	20	12	170
potatoes au gratin	⅓ of 11½ oz pkg	80	6	120
scalloped potatoes	4 oz	80	6	110
spinach soufflé	4 oz	80	9	140
yams & apples	5 oz	20	3	160
Vlasic				
Old Fashioned sauerkraut	1 oz	<20	0	4

❑ **VINEGAR** *See* SALAD DRESSINGS, MAYONNAISE, VINEGAR, & DIPS

❑ **WHEY** *See* MILK, MILK SUBSTITUTES, & MILK PRODUCTS

	Portion	Calcium (mg)	Total Fat (g)	Total Calor

❑ **YOGURT** *See* MILK, MILK SUBSTITUTES, & MILK PRODUCTS

❑ **YOGURT, FROZEN** *See* DESSERTS, FROZEN